hCGChica's
HCG DIET WORKBOOK

3 BOOKS IN 1

COACHING,
DIET GUIDE,
& PHASE 2
DAILY TRACKER

RAYZEL LAM

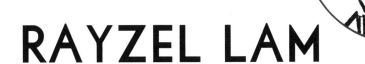

Disclaimer: This book is not intended to treat or diagnose any medical conditions. The author is not a medical professional, is not qualified to give medical advice, and is just sharing what worked from personal experience. Anyone considering this protocol should consult directly with their doctor or medical healthcare provider. The author assumes no responsbility for the use or misuse of the information in this book. Anyone doing the hCG diet does so at their own risk.

FDA required statement: The FDA has not approved the use of HCG for weight loss and reports no evidence that HCG is effective for the treatment of obesity.

Lots of free guidance and tips
for the hCG diet at:
hcgchica.com
or scan this QR code:

Gratitude TIME

DR. S.

What would we do if Dr. Simeons hadn't decided to do such interesting experimentation with the hCG hormone? Who else would have pioneered the way in such a fashion?

I'm so grateful that he discovered this and took the time to write his findings and method in his manuscript Pounds and Inches that we are continuing to benefit from, many years later.

YAM AND BEARBS

You're just going to have to guess who those people are. Just kidding. The two most important men in my life, whom I just happen to have very odd nicknames for. Not exactly sure *what* I would do without them.

FACEBOOK FANS AND THE HCGCHICA.COM EMAIL LIST

Probably sounds weird to thank an email list or a facebook page. But that's the thing. It's not just an inanimate list or page of names. There are real, down to earth helpful people that these groups are made of.

Seriously, you guys are amazing. While compiling and creating this workbook, I often turned to my facebook page to ask your feedback on what I might be missing or over-looking that you would want in such a book and received some great suggestions, many of which I have incorporated into the final draft. Those of you on my email list through my blog have been so helpful numerous times. In fact, many of the daily *hCG tips* listed on the phase 2 tracking pages are user submitted from these lovely people, sharing what kept them sane on the diet.

Aside from this, when I wanted to hear more input on an hCG related matter for my in-depth articles on the blog, I would often get 60 -100 replies, sharing very personal stories, which shows just how much we all desire to help each other out of this mire of low self worth and weight issues.

STOP!

You almost missed the

NOT-A-STINKY-SOCK THANK YOU GIFT.

What in the world is that? And if it's not a stinky sock, what IS it?

The stinky sock thing was a silly joke I started to let hCG peeps know that I had a free gift for purchasers of the workbook and that it was *a gift that had substance* and would actually help them - not some cheesy pointless gift like a dirty sock ;).

Not only was the demand for the video series HUGE, which is why I've decided to continue offering it, **I started getting emails like, "sending for my dirty sock!" and "would love a stinky sock please!"**

Boy that was great. I love that we all have a sense of humor to keep life fun.

So what is it really?

I thought you'd never ask.

> THANK YOU GIFT=
> A FREE 5 DAY
> MOTIVATIONAL VIDEO SERIES
> I CREATED JUST FOR YOU.

To get YOUR not-a-stinky-sock gift:

Just email **freegift@hcgchica.com** with any sort of proof of purchase - screenshot of your order, or hey **even a pic of your book next to your kitty will do!**

I'll reply with the 5 day video series link.

HERE'S A SNEAK PEAK
OF WHAT YOU'LL BE GETTING

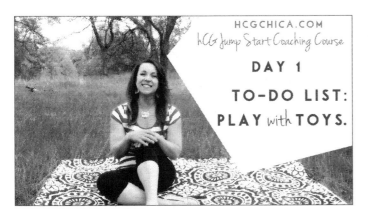

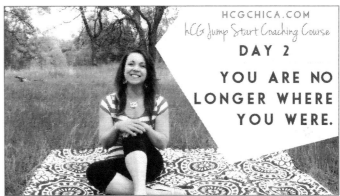

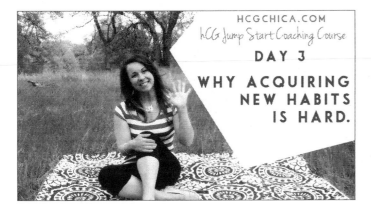

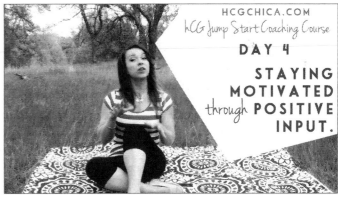

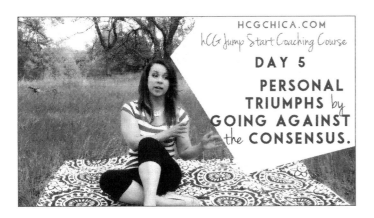

I HOPE THIS HELPS YOU GET STARTED IN A POSITIVE WAY!

Find me here:

Facebook: hcgchica | Pinterest: hcgchica
Instagram: hcgchica | Twitter: hcgchica

THERE'S A LOT HERE. YES I KNOW.

If you feel a little overwhelmed by the scope of it all,
I have a few suggestions to help you.

1. Watch my little **TUTORIAL** where you can get a visual of me showing you how you can use this workbook and let me explain and break it down with examples. **Plus you can then meet me in person**...well kinda. Through video anyway. :)

HCGCHICA.COM/P2WORKBOOK

2. When I am learning something new and I'm overwhelmed by not understanding what every other word means, let alone the whole topic, I have discovered just how amazing **SLEEP** is. Sleep really allows your body to do the work of making sense of things in your brain. If I do this continually for a few days, I find that I begin to understand a new topic much more clearly and deeply than when I first started reading about it, and in no time, I feel I understand it well.

3. Read it in **SMALL CHUNKS**. Don't try to read this entire thing in one go. Remember what we said about sleep? Read a few pages. Sleep. Read a few pages. Go to bed. Read a few pages. Sleep. You're brain is smart and will treat you well in response!

Table of CONTENTS

Section 1:

GUIDANCE FOR SUCCESS ————————— 10

Section 2:

DIET INSTRUCTIONS ————————— 54

Section 3:

QUICK GLANCE PROGRESS —————— 77

Section 4:

DAILY TRACKING AREA —————— 98

Section 5:

REFLECTIONS & PERSONAL NOTES — **249**

Section 6:

PHASE 2 CALORIE COUNT CHARTS — **262**

IF YOU CHANGE
THE WAY YOU
LOOK AT THINGS
the THINGS YOU LOOK AT
change.

- *Wayne Dyer*

Section

1

····

GUIDANCE for SUCCESS

BEHIND EVERY

ACHIEVEMENT,

large AND SMALL,

LIES A *Plan.*

– MICHAEL GORE

A Little About **HCGCHICA**

First of all, you might be wondering, WHO IN THE WORLD IS HCGCHICA? And what kind of a name is that? **C'MON SERIOUSLY.**

It was all pretty much an accident really. This whole 300 youtube videos and hcgchica.com thing.

My 5'1" frame was sitting at my desk, no doubt littered with chewed on baby stuff that belonged to my 14 month old son, in my size 16 jeans that felt like they'd been manufactured by a rubberband company, when I created my very first youtube account.

With a deep breath and nervous jitters, I was going to share my progress on the hCG diet just like I saw others doing. Oh yes of *course* I felt shy! Are you kidding? Talking to a little black square with a glass eye on my computer like it's a person? I felt so stupid! At first.

To do the whole youtube thing I had to pick a user name right? Chica just happens to be this word I used a lot in high school, like "Hi chica!" Even though I'm not Hispanic and my 3 years of Spanish in high school still left me inadequate when it comes to foreign language. hCG is self explanatory. Put 'em together, and wa-la. hCG-

Chica. Short and simple.

That was in February 2011. 300 youtube videos and 200 hcgchica.com coaching articles later, what started simply as a way to stay accountable to myself turned into a way to help others on this protocol. I've reported my findings on what seemed to work or not work when it came to having success, both with losing weight using hCG, *and* maintaining that weight loss long term, something I've been doing for over 2 years as of early 2015.

Basically, I'm just a regular person who lost about 50 pounds with the hCG diet and have been keeping it off since late 2012. I got out of those size 16 pants that were squeezing the life out of me and into a comfortable size 4, key word *comfortable!*

Lastly, I pretty much put this whole book together myself, so if my writing is a bit amateurish here and there, well, that's why. I wanted to communicate with you as the real person that I am to the heart of the real person that you are - as if you were a friend on my porch, sitting over a cup of steaming tea. Preferably hibiscus tea, it's my fav. - Rayzel

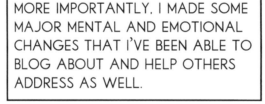

MORE IMPORTANTLY, I MADE SOME MAJOR MENTAL AND EMOTIONAL CHANGES THAT I'VE BEEN ABLE TO BLOG ABOUT AND HELP OTHERS ADDRESS AS WELL.

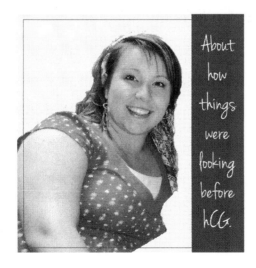

About how things were looking before hCG.

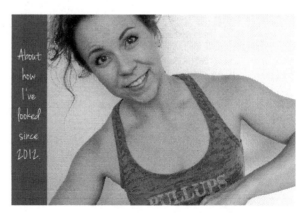

About how I've looked since 2012.

If you'd like to learn more about my personal weight loss story (and what I'm up to now!) go to **HCGCHICA.COM/MYSTORY**

Please be AWARE

· · · · ·

I am trying to pose as an expert.

Just kidding!

I am NOT an expert.

I do not have any degrees or
medical background.

I'm just sharing what I have found to work
for me personally based on trial and error
and my own personal research online.

The following ideas and suggestions are what
allowed me to stop yo-yo dieting and enabled
me to finally lose all my excess weight and
keep it off for good.

Whether this will work for you, I cannot say.
What I *can* say is we must all try and keep
seeking solutions, and I'm sharing the solutions that worked for me.

A long letter from ME to YOU

Hiya. It's me again.

You might feel scared and skeptical. Or possibly scared but hopeful. I wanted to reach out and reassure you because I started out where you are right now and I remember. It's hard to be in a place where perhaps you've tried to lose weight so many other times and it either didn't really work at all, or it worked temporarily, but didn't last.

Perhaps you even felt like *you* were the ultimate complication for why some of the approaches didn't work. I had some pretty crummy self-loathing going on for a time because I didn't seem to have the self control to do what I thought I should be doing. It was such an awful feeling to know that my choices were effecting me and hence my family in a negative way, and yet I couldn't seem to stop!

Each time these diet attempt failures happen, it feels like our self confidence has just barely survived a typhoon and we're quite a bit worse for the wear. We're alive, but pretty bedraggled. Our gifts - the things we are naturally talented at, become submerged by this low self worth. Our spirit cowers further and further inward, into this little dark hole where no one gets to *see* the talents our person has to share with the world. It becomes hard to hope because we've only experienced failure.

AND YET, ONE OF THE ONLY WAYS TO ACHIEVE A BETTER OUTCOME IS TO BELIEVE ENOUGH TO TRY SOMETHING.

I was really worried when I decided to try the hCG protocol that I would somehow be the only person to not lose weight. Somehow I would take these injections and follow this special diet, and even though everyone else I saw on youtube was losing weight, I'd get on the scale and the numbers would stay exactly the same.

My fears were unfounded. While there may be times that you experience a stall here and there (of which I've had several!) this protocol by and large allows most people to lose a significant amount of weight in a rather short period of time.

It's okay to have a wait and see attitude if you're afraid to get your hopes up. As long as you are willing to respect the guidelines of the diet enough to follow the basic set of rules,

YOU WILL BE ABLE TO ALLOW THE RESULTS TO FUEL THE FIRST CONCRETE GLIMMERS OF HOPE.

Additionally, you know how I mentioned that thing about feeling that I had no self control?

Well I also discovered along this journey that there were some very practical steps that I had to take that actually changed my ability, as if overnight, to exhibit what we might think of as will power. You'll see a few of these ideas that helped me peppered throughout the Phase 2 instructions and tips areas as well as discussed at more length on my blog, hcgchica.com

Mostly I just wish I could give you a big hug and tell you that *you are not alone.*

Whatever you weigh, right this very minute? Someone else has had the same starting weight as you, I promise.

Do you have a history of compulsively eating entire boxes of cookies or tortilla chips? So do I!

Do you have a series of chronic health issues that are numerous and confusing, some of which neither you nor your doctor really understand let alone know how to treat in a way that leaves you feeling consistently well? Believe it or not, it's true, I have dealt with this as well and I receive *frequent* emails from ladies dealing with all manner of chronic illness who are making a success of this protocol.

Out of I'm-the-only-one thoughts yet? Okay.

WE ALL START SOMEWHERE, USUALLY AT THE VERY BEGINNING, AND THAT'S OKAY.

To be honest, the triumphs you'll experience are that much sweeter and precious to you when your starting point is somewhere you didn't want to be. You can observe the progress and see where you've come from.

When I experience a new accomplishment at Crossfit, whether it's lifting a heavier weight, or gaining the strength and coordination to do a one armed handstand, the feeling of elation and satisfaction is so much more expansive given where I started. I can think back to when I hated sitting on the floor because my heaviness made getting back up so difficult. Oh the difference, the comparison!

I wouldn't feel nearly as triumphant if I hadn't first had to wade through and away from 50 lbs and made the emotional and mental changes that maintaining that weight loss shows I've made.

This precious history is what continually feeds my determination to sustain my current healthy lifestyle.

So let this be a philosophical starting point. Chronicle it for your future. Don't worry about failing. Maybe you will fail here and there along the way. It might be for a day, it might be several months.

That's okay. You don't have to be mortified that you took before photos if you fail, like it's the ultimate embarrassment, even though no one even knows you took them. I know you might be thinking this because it's what I thought. Suffering minds think alike. You don't have to be embarrassed or mortified, because you **will** be starting fresh again, as many times as it takes to succeed. Have you heard that saying? Fail your way to success? It's learning about yourself and what doesn't work for you that helps you figure out what **does** work.

That is quite literally how I was able to lose and maintain my weight loss from the hCG protocol. I discovered some things that made me fail. So I did something **different** to make things turn out better.

That is the one thing I never did previously when I tried to lose weight. I just kept trying diets, over and over, blindly, without analyzing why I failed at them.

YES, THIS CHANGE **IS** POSSIBLE FOR YOU.

And as a person whose beginning point includes watching the Biggest Loser show while eating an entire 1/2 gallon of Pralines 'N Cream, I can say that truthfully to you, even if you're covered in Oreo crumbs right now. Yes, change is possible for you.

But I'm not going to leave you hanging. The following pages will help you see *how* you can go about making these changes.

- Rayzel

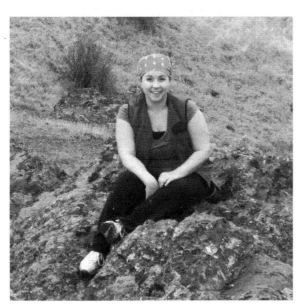

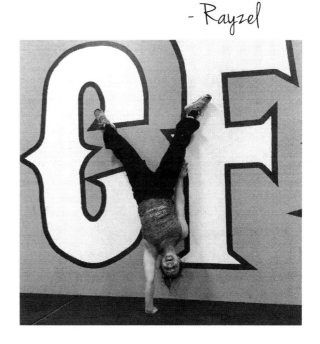

It All STARTS HERE

I developed this workbook to allow you to not only track your outer transformation during your weight loss journey with the hCG protocol, but also your inner transformation.

I've found that's what it takes to maintain weight loss. An inner change. The nice thing is that it doesn't have to happen in an instant in order to reach and stay at your goal. In fact, it *won't* happen that way. It involves forming new habits, and along the way will most likely include some mistakes, and that's okay.

By logging what you do, and how you feel, you can get to the root of what **is** working, or what **doesn't** work - for you personally.

This is what will help you navigate in a way that is tailored specifically to you, making long term success at maintaining more within reach.

HOWEVER, THERE IS ALSO A WRONG WAY TO USE THIS BOOK.

HUH? YEP.

If you find yourself over-analyzing the details and worrying excessively....over weight loss that doesn't seem to be as high as you think it should be, or inches going down slower than you feel they should, either stop doing that, or stop using this book. I mean it.

I have interviewed those who actually do *better* not tracking anything at all. So really gauge how you respond emotionally to the way you go about this and adjust either your method or yourself as needed.

These are simply tools and if you are able to detach yourself from these numbers emotionally and really use them just as tools, then I think this will be useful for you.

It might be considered a cliche to say

"THIS IS A JOURNEY"

but there's a reason this phrase is used a lot. That's really what it is! A journey. Not a one month countdown to the latest party coming up where you're distressed over being judged by your distant relatives. Oh yes, I know those anxieties.

I spent a lot of time doing that yo-yo thing. There were many reasons for it, but looking back, one of the main contributing factors is that I was always trying to lose weight for some seemingly important event in life where I'd be seen, some party or vacation. Instead of trying to lose weight for deeper reasons, with the long term in mind.

Of course I also knew I wanted to be a healthy size for me, but my efforts were not effective because I was too distracted by what for a long time was an overriding awareness of needing to look normal to other people, which led me to make poor choices about when and how I went about my weight loss. I had to get past that mentality, and then I was able to execute what I wanted to achieve all along.

There are now a number of variations of the original hCG diet plan that Dr. Simeons created.

I tried to design this workbook in a way that you could use it no matter what hCG diet method you choose to follow.

HOW TO USE *this Workbook*

I HAD A SLIGHT PANIC ATTACK when the thought struck me that you might open to the various tracking sheets here, have a flashback to your grade school days, and feel that you have to pencil something into every field and check off every box or you won't be applying yourself.

IT'S THAT WEIRD SUBCONCIOUS THING THAT PULLS FROM YOUR INNER 4TH GRADER.

Therefore, just to be clear, that is *not* the purpose of this workbook. You aren't supposed to fill out *everything*. Use the workbook to fit your unique needs.

> USE ONLY THE FIELDS YOU NEED, ALIGNED WITH HOW YOU HAVE PERSONALLY CHOSEN TO DO THIS DIET.

Since the workbook is meant to be flexible, there are some areas you may not need at all.

Examples:

CALORIES. There is a slot for calories for each food group, for each meal, and a total for each day. *This is not to suggest that you should count calories on hCG!* I didn't do so on most of my rounds, and honestly, I still wouldn't want to. It's really not necessary.

However, I realize that everyone is different. Some people feel safer or more in control counting calories, at least at this point in their journey, so that's why these fields are there; for those who find this comforting and useful. Don't count calories just because the fields are there.

Or, you may not count them *most* of the time, but then if you run into trouble on the diet and wonder if you're eating more than you think, you might count calories just for a few days to give yourself a general idea of what you've been up to.

BREAKFAST AND SNACKS. Some find that they do better breaking up their allotted 500 calories throughout the day, instead of just the lunch and dinner meals. So I created areas to easily note this. If you are one of those people who doesn't need breakfast on hCG, don't eat breakfast on hCG.

SUPPLEMENTS. If you take them, note them. If you don't, leave it blank!

LITERS VS. OUNCES. Or should I say litres? The hCG community is global folks! Don't be confused by the 2 charts for tracking liquids intake. Use whichever one makes sense to you.

HOMEOPATHIC DOSING. Most homeopathic hCG require only 3x's a day dosing and if that's working for you, stick with it. The reason I added a 4th dosing area is because some have found that their hunger was more easily managed by spreading their full homeopathic hCG daily dose into 4 doses instead of 3. So again, just making this flexible to help you be the most successful with the way you choose to approach this protocol.

OKAY, SO WE'RE GOOD ON THAT? *Moving on then.*

THE WORKBOOK: Why Flexible?

I CREATED THIS WORKBOOK IN A WAY THAT
YOU CAN USE IT NO MATTER WHAT HCG DIET
METHOD YOU CHOOSE TO FOLLOW.

Once you've done your homework, I want you to do this protocol in the way that fits best with your own personal belief system, minus your negative beliefs about yourself of course. You are an adult (I'm assuming!) You have the right to do this diet the way you deem advantageous to you.

Certainly research is in order before making such a choice. Even after doing so however, people make different decisions.

As for me, I'm somewhere in the middle on how I view what I would consider responsible when doing this diet. That's because I've had what I consider long term success with being somewhere in the middle.

There are now a number of variations of the original hCG diet plan that Dr. Simeons created. Some choose to be the experiment warriors; trying new things to see what happens. At some point, enough people having good results with the same variations leads us to believe that this particular modification is fairly reliable for yielding good results. Some choose to play it perfectly safe and follow Dr. Simeon's original protocol, exactly as it was written, to a T.

There is also what I'll call **THE SANITY FACTOR** that must be considered. Sometimes a slight deviation may be in order if it saves your sanity, doesn't appear to cause harm, and prevents you from quitting entirely.

My own choices about how I did this diet morphed from a blend of two things. One, I wanted to be sure of my results for my time spent. I don't have much

---

THE 2 EXTREMES.

"Do ONLY what Dr. S said!! Anything else and you'll fail!"

"I'm going to eat a brick of cheese on hCG and still lose weight!"

---

energy for do-overs. Two, I researched a lot to see if there was reason to believe that a particular modification would likely lead to a result just as good, or better, than the original guidelines.

Are there approaches to this protocol that I wouldn't personally do or recommend? Yes! I'm very open about my take on things on my blog. I *do* think certain methods will not only bring less than stellar results (and I am not speaking purely from a weight loss standpoint) but may even harm your body in the process. As a result, some experiments I would personally view as unwise. But part of this process is about gathering information and adapting as things become more clear.

Some start out doing the diet one way, but after further research, change their minds, and decide to approach it in a different manner. This is one advantage to providing as much information as I can to you guys through hcgchica.com. Sometimes the reason a person is using one approach is simply because they didn't have access to more helpful or accurate information initially.

To get you started, I'm going to share with you 2 methods just for reference and comparison: the original diet, as Dr. Simeons the creator of the diet wrote it, and some variations to it that I personally used in my own weight loss journey that I feel comfortable recommending. If you are following another hCG plan, by all means do that.

You can get a lot more details on following this diet successfully, as well as how to maintain weight loss, by going to hcgchica.com/diet

STAYING SANE on the hCG Diet

You don't actually have to buy a lot of stuff to do this diet - you can just get your hCG kit, grocery shop each week like usual but with your Phase 2 approved foods list and you're pretty much good.

However, most of you will soon discover that this protocol can be rather difficult to adhere to. So I'd like to share 3 useful hCG resources that many people use.

Challenge 1:
WHAT'S THE BEST STEVIA? HOW CAN I HAVE CHOCOLATE WITHOUT HAVING CHOCOLATE? AND STUFF LIKE THAT.

Solution:
Find people's favorite tips and tricks for staying sane:
HCGCHICA.COM/HCGSANITY

Challenge 2:
YOU'RE SICK OF EATING THE SAME BORING DISHES OVER AND OVER.

Solution:
TAMMY SKYE'S HIGHLY RATED GOURMET HCG COOKBOOKS.

How to Check It Out:

Left to my own creativity, I only came up with a few good recipes using the ingredients allowed.

Thankfully, there is already an amazing **chefy brain** woman out there, who did the hCG diet, and then made 2 gourmet cookbooks just for hCG.

If you are the type of person who can't handle boring, or can't handle the same meals day after day, then I highly recommend her cookbooks.

My own mother felt Tammy's cookbook was a lifesaver on the diet. She found a few favorites and made up large batches at a time and portioned them out.

Some don't mind eating the same food daily. I'm kind of like that. But for the rest of you, there's recipes.

> **Go to:**
> HCGCHICA.COM/COOKBOOKS
> to check them out and access
> <u>free recipes</u> from her book!

Challenge 3:
THIS DIET IS MORE MENTALLY CHALLENGING THAN YOU REALIZED.

Solution:
ROBIN WOODALL'S BOOK: WEIGHT LOSS APOCALYPSE – EMOTIONAL EATING REHAB THROUGH THE HCG PROTOCOL.

How to Check It Out:

Robin's book gets to the heart of some of the core issues behind our struggles with food, weight, and how we view ourselves and our body. Additionally, she talks about the **science** of this protocol, how it works, and how the hormone is interacting with our bodies. This is truly valuable because it helps us to take this protocol seriously.

> **Go to:**
> HCGCHICA.COM/HCGBOOKS
> to learn more about her book.

4 Important REALITY CHECKS

1. IT'S A HORMONE. Interacting with other hormones.

Hormones are incredibly powerful in the body. Without them you'd be dead. They are essentially the main drivers behind the multitude of functionings in our body. Tiny amounts of hormones that can be contained in small tablets are powerful enough to prevent pregnancy, to raise your metabolism and cause muscle growth.

Why some in educated circles think it's such a preposterous idea that a hormone could preserve lean muscle on a low calorie diet as well beats me, when experts accept and have proven that hormones can do many other things that are of similar caliber.

hCG is indeed a real hormone. As such it is powerful and has the potential to both positively and adversely us.

One thing to keep in mind is that hormones interact with other hormones, and this is likely true of hCG as well.

Robin Woodall, in her book *Weight Loss Apocalypse - Emotional Eating Rehab Through the hCG Protocol*, explains the theory that hCG is acting on the hormone Leptin, and that is the reason being on the *right dose* of hCG allows a person to not feel hungry on the 500 calorie diet.

What this means to me is to take this protocol seriously. We aren't simply eating less food on this diet. We're taking a hormone, that's interacting with other hormones. The choices we make on the protocol can possibly change that interaction for better or for worse.

2. These Are Theories. NOT PROVEN FACT.

It would probably take millions of dollars, tons of organized experiments and data collecting, along with proven unbiased sources who were gathering and reporting such data, to prove exactly what the hCG protocol is accomplishing.

This simply doesn't exist, and I kind of doubt ever will because there's no money in it for the big cahoonas. So really, the effectiveness of the hCG diet you could say is JUST theories. There are many accompanying factors that could be involved for why a person either has excellent long term success or fails dismally at this protocol.

I have continued to do a *lot* of healthy things for my body since ending hCG, and not only can I say it's possible these have contributed to my ability to maintain my weight, I know it has, so hCG is not the sole factor behind my long term success.

You must do your own information gathering and decide for yourself whether this protocol is worth taking a chance on or not.

3. Cheating on hCG is very COUNTERPRODUCTIVE.

You can easily take a day or two off from most diets without doing excessive damage to your overall progress.

I don't mean to scare you here, because **if** you make a mistake, it's done, so the next best thing to do is simply move on and leave guilt aside.

But if I may, I'd like to mention something that may be just enough impetous to prevent cheating on this protocol, at least sometimes!

Recall how in reality check #1 we discussed that this is a real hormone, interacting with other hormones?

Cheating on hCG seems to have more....consequences, than if you were to take the same actions (ie. eating a piece of cake or 3 beers) while not using the hCG hormone.

It can take a few days to a week to recover from a cheat. Not always, but definitely sometimes. It seems that this has to do with how the level of carbs and fats affects your body with hCG in your system. What seem to be minor indiscretions can show up on the scale as being huge blunders.

So just a warning there. Cheating on this protocol really is never worth it. Doesn't mean you won't fall victim now and again (I did) but being aware of this helps to curb the tendency to cheat or to take cheating lightly.

If it does end up happening, no need to fret. Please see *Fixing a Diet Cheat* in *Section 2 - Diet Instructions*.

4. DEBATES ON whether or not to follow the original protocol

In general, you can't really go **wrong** following the original protocol of Dr. Simeons. His protocol works. It worked then, it works now. Can you get good results with some modifications? My experience is sometimes yes. It really depends on **which** modifications you make.

The difficult thing about knowing for sure if a modification works well in your particular case is

that it's pretty much impossible to do 2 rounds of hCG under exactly the same conditions, to know if one method outperforms the other.

Ultimately, how closely you choose to follow the original protocol is a personal decision. You can make wise choices in this regard by basing that personal decision on research and discernment.

HCGCHICA.COM – RAYZEL LAM

Expected
WEIGHT LOSS

IT'S **GOOD**

TO WANT A *good outcome.*

BUT IF THESE WANTS

make you unhappy

WITH ANYTHING BUT WHAT'S UNLIKELY,

YOUR HAPPINESS WILL BE UNLIKELY TOO.

SEE IN YOURSELF INSTEAD

Achievement

BASED ON LOVE AND LOGIC.

Expected **WEIGHT LOSS**

WHILE I'M NOT A SCIENCE BUFF, I DO HAVE A FEW POINTERS THAT I BELIEVE MAKE LOGICAL SENSE TO HELP US ALL GET A SANE PERSPECTIVE ON WHAT TO EXPECT – OR RATHER, HOW TO NOT OVER-EXPECT.

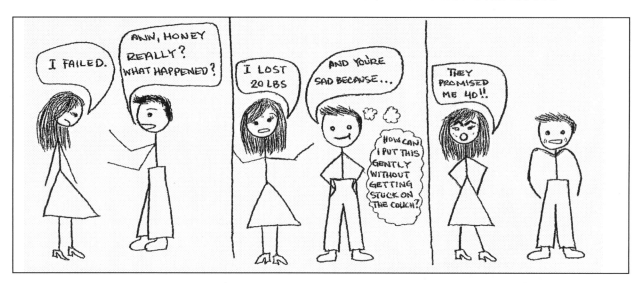

EXPECTATION POSTPONED MAKES THE HEART SICK.
– Proverbs 12:13

40 lbs in 40 days!

WE'VE ALL HEARD IT.

Do some lose this much? Yes.
But the majority do not.

First of all, no one can promise you a certain amount of weight loss. Our bodies are far too complex for that. So if someone *does* promise you a certain amount of pounds in a certain amount of days, my best advice is to just pretend you never heard it.

Over-expectation can cause a lot of problems, none of which will help you get to your goal.

It's easy for websites online to state this grand promise because it's so astounding it sells more.

There's a very logical, scientific reason that most people don't lose a pound a day that makes perfect sense.

I'd like to explain it because unrealistic expectations have led to frustration, unwise choices to try to force more weight loss, and sometimes even giving up entirely when expectations are not being met. None of these things help you arrive at your final destination and actually put you farther away from it.

Okay so lets get to it.

There's about 3500 calories in 1 pound of fat right? Many of us are familiar with this. Okay, after further research, there doesn't appear to be a very solid basis for how this number was derived. However, we can still use this as a *general* guideline.

This means that while on hCG, in order **to lose an entire pound of fat on the hCG diet every day, your body's metabolism would have to be utilizing 4000 calories every single day** (3500 calories for the pound of fat + the 500 calories you are eating each day on the diet).

The reality is I don't know too many women who utilize 4000 calories on a daily basis. In fact, I don't think I personally know *any*. The average woman appears to have a basal metabolic rate of about 1500 calories or so, you can add some calories for your various activities you do each day, and you see it's not likely to be more than 2000-2500 calories or so. That's just my guess.

It is said that the hCG hormone may raise metabolic rate a little, but it's highly unlikely that it's doubling it, wouldn't you agree?

Now in truth, some weight loss at the start of any diet is water, including hCG, and that doesn't take 3500 calories worth to lose. It's easy to drop 2-4 lbs worth of water overnight just by fasting or eating low carb. This is one reason the 1st week on the hCG protocol in particular is often so astounding when it comes to pounds lost.

So it's not necessarily that weight loss on hCG will equate to 100 percent fat.

But this fact about the requirements it takes to lose a whole pound of fat is what helps make it clear that the likelihood of the average person losing 40 lbs in 40 days or what not, is small.

Those who do are either men, very large, or both. Men do have faster metabolisms than women and have a larger calorie expenditure on a daily basis. Those who are very heavy with a lot of weight to lose likewise have a larger amount of calories that their body expends and uses to maintain their body mass. Lastly, the heavier you are and the more poorly you've been eating, the more water weight you are likely carrying. This is another reason for sometimes seeing huge drops in weight during the first week or two of hCG for those starting at a heavier weight, something not seen as much for someone with only say 20-30 lbs to lose.

AVERAGE WEIGHT LOSS FOR WOMEN ON HCG

The average weight loss for most women by the end of a long 40-ish day round is usually about .5 lb/day. If you are heavier, the average may end up being as high as .75-.80 lb per day, and if you don't have that much to lose, your average may be more like .3 lb/day.

So you may lose anywhere between 15 and 32 lbs during a 40 day round. I realize that is a big range! 32 lbs is more than twice as much as the low end of 15 lbs. What factors which number you get and is there anything you can do to make your numbers better? We'll talk about that in just a minute!

I want to clarify quickly the pattern of weight loss. When I say average of .5 lb/day, I don't mean you will lose a half pound every day on the diet. This is more how it transpires:

Some days you'll lose a lot more. Ahh those divine 1-3 lb weight loss days. Revel in those. However, obviously for the overall weight loss to average out to the .3 lb-.75 lb range, there will be some compensatory lower loss days. So you will see plenty of .2's and .4's and even big fat zero days. That is what gives you the *average* for the whole round, and this is completely normal.

AVERAGE WEIGHT LOSS FOR MEN

You might just want to skim right past this part ladies. It's just going to make you mad. Men simply lose faster. So if you're a man reading this, congrats!

It actually *is* common to have an average 1 lb/day weight loss. I still say you shouldn't expect it, because it certainly can't be counted on for every round for every man, but such results are indeed fairly typical.

WHY MEN LOSE MORE

I'm not going to claim to know the exact science behind the reason, because I don't, but a few things I've gleaned in my research are this:

More of a man's total weight is muscle than for women. What I mean by this is, if there is a man and woman and each of them weighs 180 lbs, the man's 180 lbs will usually have a much higher ratio of muscle to fat, and the woman will have more of her 180 lbs as fat. This is significant because the larger amount of muscle equates to a higher metabolism. This is just a natural fact of life. It's not because they do more squats or push-ups than you, it's part of their genetic make up.

Men have higher metabolisms, again in part due to having a large amount of fat free mass.

Testosterone levels. We all know guys have way more.

FACTORS
THAT AVERAGE WEIGHT LOSS

Short rounds (3 weeks) typically experience a higher average weight loss than long rounds (6 weeks) in part because the larger losses from the first week or two that includes more water weight than normal is averaged out over a shorter period of time. From what I've seen though, the pace of actual fat loss on hCG during short and long rounds are about the same.

Any modifications you make to the protocol like the one week pre-hCG diet and low carb loading I mention in this book may make your overall weight loss *appear* lower compared to others because you likely will have already lost water weight prior to starting hCG with these other methods. That weight normally would have come off during your first week *on* hCG. But obviously this hasn't changed your actual fat loss on the diet itself.

Lastly, when people report their weight loss online, we often have no idea if this number includes their loading gain and just how much loading weight it was. It's not uncommon for me to hear of traditional loaders (allowing sugar and carbs during the loading phase) on their 3rd or 4th round gaining 8-10 lbs during a 2 day dirty load. You can see the discrepancy there. If someone lost 30 lbs on a 40 day round, but 8 of it was loading weight, their true net loss is 22 lbs. Say you "only" lost 23 lbs in a 40 day round, but your loading weight was 1 lb because you loaded clean. Turns out your net weight loss is exactly the same as the person who seemed to have lost a lot more than you.

Some women will lose 30-35 lbs in 40 days on the diet, but this is almost always a woman with a lot of weight to lose, and from what I have seen, is not the norm, and we already discussed why earlier.

KNOWING WHAT IN THE WORLD IS GOING ON REALLY HELPS

I found learning all these details so helpful in my later rounds and it prevented me from feeling (as often anyway!) that I was doing something wrong or that my body wasn't performing on par with 'everyone else.'

I have seen the truth of the proverb quoted at the outset of this article over and over in the hCG experience when expected results are allowed to rule the person's view of their success and subsequent happiness.

The key to feeling good about your achievement on this protocol for each round you do is to stop expecting and to be pleasantly surprised with your results, whatever they may be. Each pound gone is a big achievement for your body.

When you really think about it, can someone else truly dictate for you what your body will do, in advance? You can't even do that and it's your body!

This is why it's a pitfall to put too much faith in the numbers that are thrown out there. Especially when it's not backed by any sort of logic.

Every round for you will likely be different when it comes both to total weight loss and even the pattern of weight loss.

Additionally you might discover some things along the way that slow you down, warranting the need to make corrective adjustments here and there. It could be easy to be frustrated by this process, viewing it as lost time. However this is just another aspect of the venture. There is a lot of good information out now about the hCG protocol that does make it possible to get the best out of a round, but there are still unknowns that can't always be discovered until you're actually in the trenches, doing the protocol. Some trial and error ends up being unavoidable at times. If you accept this philosophically now, you will cope and move past any seeming rough patches more quickly.

WHY LOSING LESS WEIGHT AS YOU BECOME LEANER or ALREADY DO NOT HAVE MUCH TO LOSE MAKES SENSE

Well. I found out it has to do with math, which has never been my strong suit. Actually that's not true- I *can* do it and I got A's in school, but I just don't *care* about it. But moving on, math is going to shed some light for us on weight loss. Let's use a fictitious person named **Fancy Pants**.

HCGER: MS. FANCYPANTS

ROUND	STARTING WEIGHT	IF WEIGHT LOSS WAS	EQUALS TOTAL % OF BODYWEIGHT LOST
1	200 LBS	30 LBS	15%
2	170 LBS	30 LBS	17%
		25 LBS	14%
		20 LBS	11%
3	150 LBS	30 LBS	20%
		25 LBS	16%
		20 LBS	13%
		15 LBS	10%
4	135 LBS	30 LBS	22%
		25 LBS	18.5%
		20 LBS	14%
		15 LBS	11%
		10 LBS	7%

LOSING A *larger* PERCENTAGE OF WEIGHT WITH EACH ROUND AS YOU GET SMALLER.

Que: IS THAT PROBABLE?

As you can see with this example above, that would actually be the case *if* you continued to lose the same number of pounds every successive round as you got smaller. I never thought about it this way until I ran the numbers. If you lost 30 lbs in 6 weeks at 200 lbs, that's 15% of your body weight. If you lost 30 lbs in 6 weeks at 150 lbs, that's now 20% of your bodyweight.

Why is this not going to be the norm?

Your percentage of weight loss most likely won't stay the same but will actually decrease to some degree because the metabolic rate of a heavier person is higher than a thinner person in general.

Why? Say it ain't so!

It takes more energy (and thus calories) for a heavier body to do all the same movements a thinner person does, whether it's sweating in the garden or simply putting the forks away from the dishwasher.

The Good News

The upside? When you are physically smaller, there is less surface area on your body, so smaller weight changes actually have greater effects on how you shrink visibly. Ie. a 5 lb weight loss may not be noticeable at all on a 190 lb clothed frame, but on a 130 lb frame would be quite noticeable.

WHY DOES 1/2 LB MAKES SENSE?

Remember, it's never this straight forward, but the following 2 estimates help us see why it's so unlikely for most women to lose an entire pound a day on any protocol. Those who do are likely carrying larger amounts of water weight than the average person.

Showing here on the opposite page are 2 charts with estimated BMR (basal metabolic rate) at various weights and ages for both a 5'1 and 5'6 woman. Take a second at look at it right now if you will.

What is basal metabolic rate? It's basically the number of calories your body burns in a day to keep you alive when at complete rest. *Since most of us are not vegetables, we all burn more calories than our BMR each day, but how much more varies a lot based on our lifestyle and activity level.*

Why does estimated BMR help us though?

It gives us a baseline and helps us to estimate a range of calories we actually *do* utilize on a daily basis with our unique lifestyle, whether we're at a desk job 40 hours a week, how much we exercise each week, if we walk around a lot, etc. So if your BMR is 1300 calories, your actual calories used each day once you factor in grocery shopping, digesting, walking around, exercise, etc., may be closer to 2000 calories.

THESE CHARTS HELP US TO SEE there can be a pretty large difference in how many calories a woman uses each day depending on her age, her weight, and even her height.

Based on this, it seems to reasonable to conclude that,

1). Women of various heights/weights/ages will vary in the amount of weight they lose and,

2). ultimately, we can see that to lose an entire pound of fat on any diet (barring weight loss from water weight etc.) will require more than just one day in most cases.

You might be starting to see now why blanket statements that everyone can and should be able to lose 40 lbs in 40 days, regardless of current weight, height, age, sex, or health level don't make no kinda sense people!

My 3 year old son once said something rather inspired when I tried to explain logically something he didn't want to accept.

Me: "Does that make sense son?"

My 3 year old little boy says:

"mmm....it makes *too* much sense."

Sometimes a 3 year old can speak to the heart of the matter in a way no adult can! It makes sense, but we don't want to accept it.

5'1 WOMAN – BMR (Basal Metabolic Rate) At Various Weights and Ages

WEIGHT	BMR AT AGE 30	BMR AGE 45	BMR AGE 60
200 LBS	1,565 CALORIES	1,490 CALORIES	1,415 CALORIES
150 LBS	1,338 CALORIES	1,263 CALORIES	1,188 CALORIES
125 LBS	1,224 CALORIES	1,149 CALORIES	1,074 CALORIES

5'6 WOMAN – BMR (Basal Metabolic Rate) At Various Weights and Ages

WEIGHT	BMR AT AGE 30	BMR AGE 45	BMR AGE 60
300 LBS	2,098 CALORIES	2,023 CALORIES	1,948 CALORIES
250 LBS	1,871 CALORIES	1,796 CALORIES	1,721 CALORIES
200 LBS	1,644 CALORIES	1,569 CALORIES	1,494 CALORIES
175 LBS	1,531 CALORIES	1,456 CALORIES	1,381 CALORIES
150 LBS	1,417 CALORIES	1,342 CALORIES	1,267 CALORIES

Remember, you DO burn more calories each day than these charts show.

This is just that "basal" or bottom-layer thing. From my research, it looks like BMR is typically about 60-70% of your actual daily calorie expenditure. So what this means is, the calories you burn total each day is likely 30-40% higher than your basal metabolic rate. So if your BMR was 1400 calories for instance, then 30% more (420 more calories) would be a total daily calorie burn of 1820 calories.

But it could be more than 40% too! This is just an example. How many calories individuals burn each day greatly varies. It depends on your activity level and the nature of your daily life. My husband is gardener and probably walks about eight miles a day while mowing lawns and chopping down trees, so he is obviously utilizing a LOT more calories in a day than someone who works at a desk.

WHY IT'S *Good* TO NOT LOSE TOO FAST

When you start tweaking with everything under the sun, my concern is that if the modifications made aren't wise, "extra" weight loss could be coming from muscle.

We can't even begin to understand the complexities of how our bodies utilize calories (or lack of them!) really.

I believe wholeheartedly in how well this protocol can work, within the principles of how it's designed. Once you go outside those principles though, there is a higher margin for negative effects.

What's difficult is that simply losing more pounds on a scale doesn't tell you *what* you are losing.

So just keep this aspect in the back of your mind when deciding whether or not to try something different on this protocol.

Remember what your true aim is and what is a reasonable amount of weight loss to expect based on what we've discussed.

WHEN HEALTH COMPLICATIONS AFFECT WEIGHT LOSS

Hormone levels. Sigh.

I can't go into all the details on this here, first of all because I'm really not educated enough to put it in book form, but also because it would take one fat book to contain it all!

However, I feel it's so important to mention because I have seen first hand just how drastically our balance of hormones can affect both ability to lose weight and to maintain weight loss. There may indeed be times when it does appear that your body is not responding well to your responsible efforts.

What I'd like to do is give you my absolute favorite online resources and current books to aid you in your personal research in finding answers to the conundrums in your own body.

These are some of the main hormones that have a huge bearing on weight and how your body utilizes calories:

- Adrenal hormones, specifically
  Cortisol and
  DHEA
- Thyroid hormones
- Progesterone
- Estrogen
- Testosterone

Use those as keywords to do your google searching.

Both too much and too little of these various hormones can cause weight gain even when you have an otherwise healthy lifestyle.

The following are what I feel to be the most useful resources to me in learning how to fix and tweak what's wrong in my body when it comes to hormones.

You can get quick links to the following resources by going to **hcgchica.com/hormonelinks** (also I keep the above link updated with new resources).

WEBSITES:

Stopthethyroidmadness.com
Jeffreydachmd.com

BOOKS:

1. **STOP THE THYROID MADNESS** - by Janie A. Bowthorpe, M.Ed.

2. **IODINE – WHY YOU NEED IT, WHY YOU CAN'T LIVE WITHOUT IT** by David Brownstein, M.D.

3. **HYPOTHYROIDISM** - Type 2 - Mark Starr, M.D.

Find links to these books at:
Hcgchica.com/hormonelinks

EH, I ALREADY HAD LAB TESTS DONE & EVERYTHING WAS NORMAL.

The two questions to ask here are, your results were normal based on what information? And specifically what tests were run?

Before I leave this topic can I pretty please **plead** with you not to end your search without first making sure you have unturned multiple stones.

Just to give you an idea of what I mean, so many end up suffering for much longer than necessary because one unhelpful test was run that showed their thyroid levels were "normal" when in actuality, if the right testing had been done, a hypothyroid condition **would** have been uncovered.

I had no idea that the general thyroid panels commonly done rarely unconver anything. More specific testing panels that are better able to pinpoint real thyroid issues are available. However, the caveat is it's very uncommon to be given these tests unless you specifically ask for them. There are so many medical advancements going on, and not all medical personnel are up to speed yet, so it really pays to do your own research and share with them what you need.

I'll give you an example. The TSH test is a general thyroid test often done. The normal reference range for TSH lab values was re-evaluated several years ago by whoever makes the guidelines for this in the medical industry. Thousands who were considered to have a normal thyroid under the old reference range for so many years prior, who were

no doubt being tested and told they were normal even though they felt awful, would now be considered hypothyroid and get treatment. That's why we can only put so much faith in testing. Symptoms **must** be part of the decision making process.

I had symptoms for years, all the while my thyroid levels were "normal." Finally my condition got so bad that my hypothyroid issue finally did show up on the standardly issued testing.

But I can put two and two together. The symptoms I had all along when the generic testing said my thyroid was "normal" were exactly the same (just not quite as severe) as when the testing finally revealed something being sorely wrong. The symptoms were not caused by two different conditions. I could have been treated much sooner had I known about the other testing because it would most likely have revealed a problem much earlier. The websites and books I have mentioned here will help you learn specifically what testing to ask for.

The only way to find out about this stuff and get help now instead of 15 years from now is by making it your personal responsibility.

Another example. My saliva cortisol levels on my lab test looked fairly normal. They were a bit low-ish but still in the reference range and would be considered normal enough by a medical office to do nothing about it. I did have adrenal fatigue symptoms however.

How did I happen to realize that I did indeed need adrenal support? Yes, reading an article online. I found the experience of a woman on stopthethyroidmadness.com who shared her saliva cortisol lab values, which were almost *exactly* the same as mine and she expressed how she felt much better after adding in a physiological dose of cortisol (even though such values were technically "in" the reference range = she was healthy enough) and that she was able to optimize her thyroid medication after doing this as well and described great symptom improvement over a sustained period of time.

I decided to follow her example and did the same. I too experienced significant improvement in my symptoms over several months. Additionally during this time I lost about 3-4 pounds of fat and gained about 3 pounds of muscle (results gathered from hydrostatic body fat testing), even though my actual lifestyle didn't change whatsoever. It appears my body was sorely needing that cortisol.

While I understand there can be hype online and that you can't put your ultimate faith in every single word written on the internet, I feel it has done people like me a lot more good than harm from the truths that I would never otherwise have uncovered on my own and that some medical personnel are not aware of yet at this time.

I'm collecting resources for finding doctors who are up to speed with current hormone testing and treatment methods that you can work with on these types of issues (and if you are such a doctor, please contact me! hcgchica@hcgchica.com):

Hcgchica.com/findadoc

I hope it's clear that I'm not recommending that people just start taking stuff. I think it's wise to get lab testing, but do that research to discover just what types of testing you need to request, do research to help interpret those lab results, then do more research on the best current treatments for those conditions.

NO ONE HAS A MORE VESTED INTEREST IN YOUR WELL BEING THAN YOU. REMEMBER THAT.

When you care, you will do whatever it takes to get to the bottom of what's wrong in your body. No one else is going to care as much you will - not your doctor, not your endocrinologist. They can help, and you may need them, but when solutions are not being found, when standby treatments are not working, the only person who will care enough and have the circumstances to spend six hours researching thyroid issues and iodine till three a.m. will be you, because you're the only person who has to live with the symptoms every moment of your life. This is not a criticism of others. It's just a truth that we have to take that responsibility for our health at a core level if we want to get the best treatment for ourselves.

Several alternative doctors have been quite helpful to me. Each one of them helped me to put together a piece of the puzzle. No one person has known all the pieces. And that's okay. It's up to me to pursue my own best health.

IDEAL BUT POSSIBLY NOT PLAUSIBLE SCENARIO:

I suppose the absolute ideal scenario would be to figure out all these hormone issues before hCG, get things all as level as possible, and then proceed with your weight loss. However, this process of balancing hormones can take a long time!

Honestly, I think it's technically probably never done in the sense of being over, because our bodies are constantly in a state of flux as we age and go through different circumstances in life. Additionally, there are costs involved with this process as well. It's not always feasible to try to do it all at once.

REALISTIC FOR NOW SCENARIO:

The truth is we only have so much time, we only have so much energy, and we only have so much brain processing power at one time.

Being real, delving into the world of what's wrong with you in relation to this hormone thing can be a bit of a tangled web. It's worth unraveling, but it requires some time and patience.

If you are already starting hCG, it may be something to look into more between rounds.

In the meantime, yes, perhaps you will have a slightly lower average weight loss than some who either have their thyroid intact or who have already gone through five doctors and two years of frustration to find adequate and ideal thyroid and adrenal support.

But really, what's the alternative? The task of addressing everything at once is often not feasible. You have to be able to make one or two small changes when it comes to fixing hormone issues and seeing how it s your symptoms, before making other adjustments. Otherwise you may feel different, better or worse, but you'll have no idea which of the many changes you made caused it, so you won't be any farther along!

That's why I feel in many cases it may be best to....

DO WHAT IS DO-ABLE FOR YOU AT THIS TIME.

I've dealt with chronic illness that has major ebbs and flows when it comes to the severity of symptoms for several years now, before, during, and after the hCG protocol.

Even though I didn't have the ultimate cause nor the ultimate cure at any time, I made it through my hCG journey amidst it all, and along the way continued to pursue discovering the imbalances in my body and how they could be corrected.

If I had waited until I felt completely "healed" or "well", I'd still probably be waiting to do my first round of hCG because to this day I continue seeking and discovering answers to some symptoms. Which means I'd still be 50 lbs overweight and living on ice-cream, certainly not something that would have been helping my long term health these past few years.

I'm quite happy with losing 27 lbs in 42 days my first round, with 20 lbs another round, and with 17 lbs in 40 days my final round. Could I have lost more if my hormones were perfect? Maybe. I'll never know. But I just wasn't able to get that all figured out at the time, so I decided to take the 20 lbs, be happy, and not worry about an extra few pounds I may or may not have lost if I had the inner workings of a perfect body. Maybe I had to spend a few extra days on hCG than someone else to get to my goal. So what? In the grand scheme of things does this really matter?

I have to go back to how strongly our mental and emotional outlook on the whole process seems to be for dictating the ultimate outcome.

You could compare the length of my journey with the false perceptions of rapid weight loss we've discussed and feel my pace was too slow, perhaps not worth it. It's important to look at the ultimate outcome however. Since I'm happy with how things transpired and accepted the pace; didn't over-analyze everything from a negative viewpoint and kept my spirits up (in general!), I stuck to what I had chosen to do on the protocol, reached my goal, and stayed there.

> **WHEN YOU ALLOW FRUSTRATION**
> and how you think things *should* be
> **TO RULE YOUR STATE OF BEING,**
> you lose so much power that
> the control you *do* have
> over your outcome can change.
> **EMOTIONAL DECISIONS CAN ENSUE**
> that are not the right ones.

If I had not done the research to see what was truly normal and expected when it comes to weight loss on hCG, I have no doubt my discouragement would have caused me to keep calling it quits on each new try.

Again, it's perception. 20 lbs is a lot you guys! If you accomplish that in 40 days, that's amazing! It's the *perception* that you were supposed to somehow attain 40 that makes 20 lbs seem dismal.

Also keep in mind that it seems that the percentage of weight lost as fat may be greater than other diets that also have fast weight loss in mind. A 20 lb weight loss on hCG may very well not be the same as a 20 lb weight loss on a plain old 1000 calorie diet with no hCG. If more of your total weight loss is fat and not something else, this means you will physically shrink *more* for the same pounds lost compared to other diets. This is just another factor to take into consideration.

Stalls on the HCG DIET

GOAL WHEN STALLS OCCUR IN PHASE 2:

MAINTAIN A BALANCE BETWEEN RESPECTING THE NATURAL PROCESS OF NON-LINEAR WEIGHT LOSS AND INVESTIGATING POSSIBLE CAUSES AND REMEDIES FOR THE STALL.

When weight loss seems to slow, or stalls completely for a number of days, paranoia can set in. **What do we do when we are are freaked out over something?** We usually make decisions based on emotion instead of logic, and that's where everything goes all poopoo-caca.

You think to yourself, oh. my. goodness. I didn't lose weight today. I'm stalling!! Ahhhhh!!! Quick, maybe I should do an apple day, or a modified steak day, or burn 500 calories on the treadmill and *make* my weight loss start back up.

If that's you, don't worry, I had a few bouts of this type of thinking as well. My very first time on the diet I didn't know what to expect or the logic behind anything. It seemed reasonable to think if I was eating only 500 calories every day, that I should lose a lot of weight every day.

The morning of day 13 on the very low calorie diet during my first round of the diet, I experienced my first day of no weight loss. A big fat zero on the scale. I ran to youtube with my sob story. "I'm in a stall guys, I didn't lose weight today...woa is me, what do I do about it?" Essentially the answer from the hCG youtube tribe at the time was, nothing. It's not a stall. It's normal to not lose weight some days. Just let it be. True stalls last for several days, and even those can be normal and may not really necessitate grand intervention.

It didn't occur to me that some days I was experiencing way *more* weight loss on the scale than could have possibly been accomplished in just one day of calorie restriction on the diet and that at some point there was going to have to be some balancing out time.

My records show that my overall weight loss as of that day was 11.6 lbs in 12 full days on the diet, with only a .8 loading gain. So almost all of it was net weight loss. In reality my average daily weight loss in the 12 day period was super high so far! But there I was all worried.

So let's address this from the logical side as to why stalls are often normal, then we'll talk about possible causes we *can* identify to see if there truly is something amiss that's fixable to allow better weight loss.

THE LEFT BRAIN LOOK AT WEIGHT LOSS ON HCG

What I came to realize is that our bodies don't behave like calculators. Weight loss is just not that predictable.

If we lose 2 lbs one day, we rejoice, but then when we lose .2 the following day, we think something is wrong. We forget to put two and two together and realize, ah! My body is either catching up or evening out etc. because there's no way I could have burned 7000 calories worth of fat in one day to yield such a 2 lb loss overnight. Some of that 2 lbs resulted most likely from what I was doing a few days prior on the diet, water weight, or both.

The results of what we do each day don't always seem to appear immediately the next morning in time for our daily scale check in. Your body doesn't care about your daily weigh in. It cares about keeping things balanced and can't usually be rushed just because you have a scale appointment. I know, bummer.

I learned to relax my view and my resulting perception of whether or not my progress on the diet was good after grasping this concept:

WEIGHT LOSS IS A LITTLE MORE ORGANIC IN NATURE AND NOT QUITE SO MECHANICAL.

You want to know why this reality based perception is important to come to grips with? In a state of expectations not being met, we will often do one of two things.

1. Give up
2. Decide to force it by making choices that may not be in our body's best interests.

THE POWER EXPECTATION HAS OVER US

Since it's probably too late and you've already read somewhere that this diet produces a pound a day of weight loss, you might have to spend a few minutes moping around and feeling sorry for yourself. Go ahead, it's okay!

I remember feeling a little let down when I realized why most people won't logically lose a pound of fat a day. That really bummed me out because that idea had been presented to me as something attainable and it was very desirable. I had already envisioned how far I would get in a short amount of time. I didn't really want to recalibrate.

It's kind of like if you heard someone was going to give you fifty grand. You got all excited about it, planning what you were going to do with it, maybe a few trips to exotic places, or building an addition on to the house. But then a few days later after you've already planned and dreamed that fifty thousand away, you found out you were mistaken, the amount was actually 25k not 50k.

You *know* it's absolutely silly to feel deflated. I mean, c'mon, someone's *giving* you money. But you can't help it - you *do* feel deflated that it's "only" twenty-five thousand dollars. If you'd never been misled to think it was fifty grand in the first place, you'd have been over the moon happy about twenty-five thousand dollars and you would have planned appropriate dreams in your head based on that.

Your expectation level would be matched with what you were going to recieve so your contentment level and emotional happiness with it would be high.

Let's say you knew it was twenty-five thousand dollars all along. You're super happy about it. Then say that same person decided to surprise with an additional three thousand dollars. Well, then you'd just be ecstatic! Feeling content and ecstatic about something positive in your life is a great recipe for making further good choices.

You want to create that scenario for yourself on this protocol. You want to expect nothing essentially (because believe me you *will* achieve weight loss, you're just not quite sure how many pounds), and then be really satisfied inside when you're on the diet and you lose whatever weight you lose.

Now let's contrast that. If you start a round of hCG with a high level of expectation, that you *must* lose 30 or 40 pounds in 40 days, the likelihood of being sorely let down is very high. Almost certain in fact, I'd say. When your spirits are low, everything feels hard. The diet feels more cumbersome, you feel like quitting, you feel like cheating, you feel like each day isn't worth what you're getting out of it on the scale.

That is *not* a recipe for doing well in the long run.

Don't confuse lowering expectations with being lax in putting forth effort to stick to the protocol though. I'm not talking about not caring here. **I'm speaking of caring in a guided way based on logic.**

That is the recipe for really making this protocol work for you.

Take the protocol seriously and know that you will achieve good results, but don't predetermine for your body what that actually equates to in pounds.

USE A BALLOON-IN-THE-SKY VIEW

Whenever you feel anxious about the pace of your weight loss, and all those .2's and .4's are really getting under your skin, step back and calculate your total weight loss in number of days on the diet.

Remember, if it's day 14, your current total weight loss is how much you've lost in 13 days, since day 14's results won't be known till the following morning.

TOTAL LBS LOST IN # OF DAYS COMPLETED ON DIET

One you have this, compare it to what we've learned about expected weight loss on the diet in the last article. Think about how many calories your body likely burns per day in your daily life, somewhere in the 1500-2500 calorie range most likely right?

Remind yourself that it takes 3500 calories to burn through a pound of fat, give or take. Then breathe. Take a moment to be irritated that it takes so many calories to get rid of that yellowy gelatinous stuff. Breathe again. Get philosophical about it. Realize you can't change science, and move on carrying your more realistic mindset in place.

FACTORS THAT COULD BE ING THE SCALE THAT DON'T REALLY MATTER:

» BATHROOM ISSUES: It's common to have fever bowel movements simply because you're eating far less than usual. Less going in = less coming out. I know, I know, this didn't occur to me either when I was new to the diet. Who can blame us? How many of us ever ate so little on a daily basis before? Sometimes it might build up over a few days until there's enough there to fuel the peristalsis/time to evacuate feeling in your body.

» EXTRA SALT: I kid you not, I had soup one night on hCG and I gained 2 lbs the next morning. I like my food fairly salted and since the volume of soup is rather large - all that liquid - when you salt it to taste, you often end up consuming more sodium than you might have otherwise. The water retention from sodium intake is temporary. I purposefully chose to eat soup daily when doing hCG during the fall/winter so that I would have what you might call a baseline for water retention. Essentially, after having one gain from salt intake, by keeping my salt intake about the same from that point forward (i.e. having soup daily), I didn't experience further weird fluctuations.

» EXERCISE: Exercise can actually cause fluid retention too. Even a simple evening walk can do this. It's nothing to worry about, but I was amazed how I could almost count on a zero loss on the scale the next morning if I took a walk around the neighborhood with my hubby the night before.

FACTORS THAT TRULY COULD BE HAMPERING YOUR WEIGHT LOSS:

» DOSE/HUNGER: Knawing hunger outside of meal times or continuing hunger outside of the 500 calories or so is usually an indication that your dose of hCG isn't adjusted to your needs. I don't feel comfortable discussing dosage in detail here, but please see my article regarding this at hcgchica.com/dosage to see what has worked well for others. I believe that if your hCG dosage isn't optimized to your unique body, the resulting hunger is an indicator that your body is not operating as well as it could on the protocol. I feel adjusting this for the proper low/no-hunger effect will aid in better weight loss overall. Technically dosage is something that must be decided by a medical professional, so please know this is simply my opinion. I don't believe there is a one size fits all in this area.

» SLEEP: Lack of both quality and quantity. There was actually a small study* done where all the

---

* Study: *Insufficient Sleep Undermines Dietary Efforts to Reduce Adiposity.* Arlet V. Nedeltcheva, MD; Jennifer M. Kilkus, MS; Jacqueline Imperial, RN; Dale A. Schoeller, PhD; Plamen D. Penev, MD, PhD. Source: annals.org October 2010|Annals of Internal Medicine|Volume 153|Number 7

participants were on the same exact diet, but half the group had their sleep restricted to 5.5 hours while the other half got a full 8.5 hours. While both groups lost about the same amount of scale weight, *the group whose sleep was restricted lost 60% more muscle than those who slept the 8.5 hours.* Which means even though the scale weight *looked* the same, in reality, a lot less of the sleep deprived group's weight loss was fat. Additionally that same group experienced both a lower resting metabolic rate and higher hunger levels. Lower metabolic rate = less weight loss, and I think you already know what higher hunger levels equal. I'm relating this to show how much sleep can have a bearing on this process for us. I'm a night owl and it's hard for me stop living and go to bed but reading this study sure is motivating isn't it!

If you're having trouble sleeping while on the diet, you can go to hcgchica.com/sleep for troubleshooting ideas.

» WATER INTAKE: Drinking enough water is an important part of this process. I think you already know the general reasons why, so I'll give you an example you may not have thought of. From my research the liver is 85-95% water. Toxins are stored in fat. When you lose fat on this diet, these toxins can be released into your bloodstream, which your liver then processes to detoxify you and get them out of your system. From what I've read, the viscosity of your blood, which is affected by how hydrated or dehydrated you are, can impact your liver's detoxification capabilities as it's filtering your blood. I feel this can affect weight loss because our bodies are always trying to protect us from toxins, so if the mechanism for getting rid of toxins is compromised, it seems likely that our bodies will hold on to both water and fat more readily.

» STRESS: Hormones are so powerful! When we refer to it as stress, it somehow seems like a non-medical thing that can't really our body, but it's just the opposite! Stress does things like raise cortisol levels. Chronically elevated cortisol can totally inhibit and prevent weight loss and even cause fat gain. Google that one, it's easy to find proof of this.

» FOOD SENSITIVITIES: It may be hard to explain the exact mechanism behind it, but many have discovered certain Phase 2 foods, unique to them, cause their bodies to stall. For some it's beef, for others cabbage, or tomatoes - it really varies. If there are Phase 2 foods you are eating on a consistent basis and you are experiencing a stall, it doesn't hurt to change it up and remove something that could be causing you issues.

» EXERCISE: Some may disagree with me on this. I'm not saying it's bad for everyone on hCG. But what I have found is that depending on your state of health when you begin this protocol, doing too many things on hCG can be like asking too much of your body at one time which seems to cause a mutiny. This diet is a full time job for your body already. I think of this protocol as a cleanse, and it's common on a cleanse for more rest than usual to be recommended. If you're adrenals and thyroid are intact, you may be able to add exercise and do quite well. However, if you are in some type of weakened state (and you may be unaware of this), the exercise and eating only 500 calories a day for several weeks *may* be too much of a strain and your body may start to resist you.

When to ALLOW Failure

I'm going to continue getting even more real with you now. I feel it's important because it's the realization that failure happens and allowing it at times that will ultimately help you reach your goal.

I know, I know. That sounds backwards. I thought so too until I finally discovered that my perception of failure was actually perpetuating failure for me over and over again.

There were two negative outcomes from my previous view of screw ups. There were two *positive* outcomes when I acknowledged and embraced my setbacks. And there is one secret I had to learn to make those positive outcomes a reality.

I'd like to share them here because I think many of you may be dealing with a similar way of processing things.

PROBLEM #1:

> Thinking failure doesn't happen to others, only to me, which must mean I'm essentially a loser.

PROBLEM #2:

> Thinking #1 leads me to either give up entirely, OR make further attempts, without changing how I go about it, leading me to the same result again; failure.

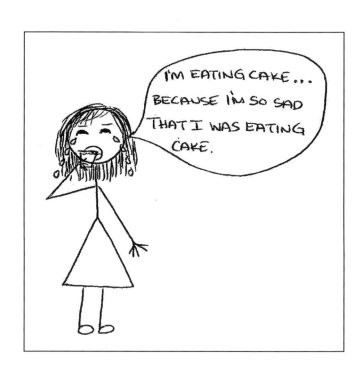

PROBLEM #1:

Thinking failure doesn't happen to others, only to me, which must mean I'm essentially a loser and my future weight loss efforts are doomed.

WHY THIS IS A FALSE BELIEF

We all screw up. When you see someone who is a success in some way, all we are seeing is where they are *now* and we tend to assume that they reached that place without failure. We do not have the full scope of how they achieved their success.

I want you to do me a favor if you tend to think this way. Go to google and look up "successful people who failed first."

You will find a myriad of people from all walks of life who became actors, business people, inventors, musicians, novelists and they all have multiple what might be considered "failures" before being recognized in some way.

It might be easy to think that these individuals are somehow part of a special elite minority of super-humans and that the majority of us can't achieve the same thing.

This isn't true. The thing is, we are *all* having small triumphs on a daily basis even now. Perhaps at the moment your relationship with food and your body isn't the best. But if you take a look at other aspects of your life, there is at least one challenge that you are meeting and rising above. Whether it's caring for an elderly parent, cooking dinner for your children even though you're exhausted, applying yourself at school or handling the many varied situations that secular work often presents.

Your ability to think about and meet challenges in small ways in your daily life means you have the means within you to meet other challenges that may seem overwhelming to you at the moment.

I'll use myself for an example. I've maintained my weight loss for over 2 years as of late 2014 and yet, I totally did fail at the hCG diet before. Bet ya didn't know that eh? My 2nd round on the protocol was an utter flop, and what is more, I spent about 9 weeks *following* my failed round living on ice-cream and cookies again. I gained back almost all the weight I lost during that 2nd round.

The round itself was a disaster, even though I *did* lose some weight, because I didn't carry it out responsibly at all, which left me feeling really crummy, was emotionally damaging to me, and I was just plain miserable for weeks on end. Constant cheating then trying to fix it. Hoping to do better the next day, but then repeating my poor choices again anyway. Over and over.

PROBLEM #2:

Thinking #1 led me to either give up entirely, OR make further attempts without changing how I went about it, leading me to the same result again; failure.

THE PROBLEM WITH PROBLEM #2:

Isn't the chocolate cake cartoon so true? I'm pretty certain if we had a room full of 100 women and asked how many of us have eaten something we'd consider not healthy in response to feeling bad over eating something else unhealthy, probably at least 75% of us would raise our hands.

But the problem with how we view ourselves when we make what we consider to be a poor choice is that this negative outlook makes us feel so discouraged, so bad about ourselves, that we don't see a way out. The best comfort in moments like these seems to be more cake or chips. We don't need to dwell on why this isn't logical because it doesn't matter! The truth is, that is simply the reaction that many of us women have.

Really, it's not so much that we ate the food itself, but more our feeling of lack of control over being able to prevent ourselves from eating _____ (insert typical go-to junk food). Also the projection of future lack of control.

The other drawback with seeing ourselves in such a condemnatory way after a poor choice is that we don't think to wonder what might be wrong with either the protocol or the approach. Instead we are focused solely on "what is wrong with ME?"

Nothing is wrong with you. It's actually the protocol, your approach, or both; but it's something fixable. You won't be free to consider this if you view a setback as an inherent inability on your part.

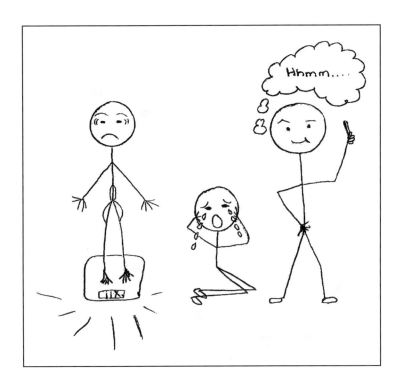

SOLUTION #1:

Give myself grace for things that didn't work out.

SOLUTION #2:

Doing #1 allowed me to feel good enough about myself to trouble-shoot the failures logically so I could avoid repeating them next time.

SOLUTION #1:

Give myself grace for things that didn't work out.

This may fall under the realm of psychology. If that's true, so be it. All I know is, for the type of personality I seem to have, this approach works for me.

The most important thing I can be given, that gives me the strength to persevere whether it's right now or a little later, is the permission to choose; to fail even.

Permission to fail takes the feeling of loss of control or the feeling that something outside myself is pressuring me to do something and makes me feel that *I* have the choice.

Why is this such a big deal?

This permission often inspires me to continue, of my own volition.

PERMISSION IS EMPOWERING IN A VERY POSITIVE, BENEFICIAL WAY. Sometimes that permission may indeed cause you to fail, for now. That's okay. But it can allow that failure to happen in a way that produces less guilt and gives you the strength to proceed with solution #2......

SOLUTION #2:

Giving myself acceptance and permission allowed me to feel good enough about myself to troubleshoot the failures logically so I could make a plan aimed at success for next time and avoid repeating that same setback.

When something doesn't work out, there can be a variety of reasons for it. **If you don't troubleshoot these, it can lead to repeating the same mistakes over and over.**

So if you do a round of hCG and it's just a total mess for whatever reason, or after the diet is a total mess, step back and and analyze logically, asking yourself these main questions:

WHAT WENT WRONG? What did I struggle with?

WHAT ARE POSSIBLE CAUSES FOR THE STRUGGLES I HAD?

HOW CAN I AVOID THESE ISSUES IN THE FUTURE? WHAT SPECIFICALLY CAN I CHANGE TO HAVE BOTH A DIFFERENT EXPERIENCE AND OUTCOME?

Note: This can't be just "I'll try harder". That is not an actionable plan. These have to be *specific* changes you are going to make.

The answers to these questions are found usually through 3 steps:

- thought
- research online
- more thought based on your research

After identifying the problems, you research what can counteract or prevent those problems.

A REAL EXAMPLE
OF HOW TO DO THIS

not like Ms. fancypants - she was pretend.

To give you an example, I will share with you my own process of doing this after my failed Round 2. The reason I'm sharing it is because it actually worked!

ME: WHAT DID I STRUGGLE WITH? WHAT WENT WRONG?

1. I struggled with very intense sugar cravings.

2. I felt depressed and very tired during the round.

3. I thought I could get away with eating strange off-protocol foods (we're talking fiber cookies with lots of sugar alcohols in place of my vegetables) thinking it wouldn't affect me; a kind of head in the sand sort of thought process.

4. When Phase 3 came, I was so burnt out because I was feeling so crappy that I stopped caring entirely. So I just ate whatever I felt like eating. I gave up and in.

ME: WHAT ARE THE MAIN POSSIBLE CAUSES FOR THE STRUGGLES I HAD?

1. I had been eating very clean for about 3 months prior to loading for my 2nd round of hCG. But when I loaded, I chose to go ahead and eat sugary foods again, as well as load for 3 days - this means for 3 days I was eating large amounts of sugar and carbs, several of which were my previous trigger binge-eating foods. I didn't feel the same after this. I had not been craving anything sugary, or felt the desire to binge in 3 months, but after I loaded in this manner, my brain suddenly felt very different and I felt a strong urgency to continue bingeing and getting my hands on large amounts of sugary foods.

I continued to have a lot of cravings on the actual 500 calorie portion of the diet and I surmised to myself that with the current state my body was in, anything containing sugar at that point (even if normally healthy) like the Phase 2 fruits, were continuing to fuel those cravings while on the diet.

2. My health was obviously in a different place than when I did my first round, looking back on it.

My chronic illness symptoms had been acting up and this made the diet feel very hard because I was really imbalanced in some way physiologically.

3. I got cocky after my first round. I remember wondering to myself if all the rules associated with the diet really mattered that much. I thought perhaps things didn't need to be as strict as I had read.

4. I allowed myself to struggle for too long when my body clearly wasn't ready for that process at that particular time, as well as doing unhealthy things on the diet itself. These two things pretty much put me at the snapping point by the time Phase 3 came around. I feel I actually should have aborted the round early.

ME: HOW CAN I AVOID THESE ISSUES IN THE FUTURE? WHAT SPECIFICALLY CAN I ALTER TO HAVE A DIFFERENT EXPERIENCE AND OUTCOME?

Note to self: Do research

PROBLEM & SOLUTION 1: I realized it was definitely a mistake to think that I could eat sugary foods, especially the ones that were my previous binge triggers, when I loaded, or at any other time really. In future, I would no longer do that. The experience taught me an important lesson.

There is never a good enough reason to over-indulge in such foods, for me personally. Me thinking that it was warranted because, 'it *is* the loading phase after all!' was me deceiving myself.

In researching the purpose of loading in Dr. Simeons original protocol, I saw that **the principle was really just that the foods be high in fat.** I reasoned this could be done without sugar being involved. Going forward I would load for the hCG protocol low carb/no sugar/high fat as a trial and see if it produced good results.

PROBLEM & SOLUTION 2: Being honest with myself, I realized that deciding to load for three days instead of two was for me not because it was needed but because I was looking for a reason to eat my favorite junk food one more day. No more decieving myself next time. The purpose in my doing the hCG protocol was to turn my life around, not to find ways to still continue my previous bad habits. I planned to load only 2 days the following round.

PROBLEM & SOLUTION 3: I googled things like "quickest way to get over withdrawal symptoms when starting a low carb diet." I knew I would most likely experience similar withdrawal symptoms trying to get off sugar again. It's those withdrawal symptoms that are a crucial time period when the likelihood of giving in is greater than at any other time.

I came across the guidance in my research that having a high fat diet during this time period, not *just* low-carb, was a crucial part of making the withdrawal symptoms go away faster as well as making them feel less acute while it was going on.

This obviously couldn't be implemented on the 500 calorie diet portion of hCG since fats are not eaten during this time. I also reasoned that going through sugar detox at the same time as only being able to eat 500 calories (essentially elminating almost all ways of "comforting" myself to get through the rough patches by being able to eat more of something else), wouldn't likely go together too well.

This gave me the idea to spend 7-10 days **prior** to starting my next round of hCG, eating not just low carb but **high fat, completely removing all sugar sources from my diet, including fruits**, at that time, to see if I could get myself past the initial hump of sugar withdrawals before starting hCG. This had the potential to make my actual experience on hCG feel much easier.

PROBLEM & SOLUTION 4: I also knew from a prior experience of trying to get off sugar, that even healthy sugars fueled my sugar cravings during the initial period of removing it from my diet.

Way before hCG, I attempted to distance myself from my sugar addiction. My approach at that time was to eliminate all refined sugar sources and grains, but to still eat whole fruits freely. I did this for about 3 weeks and I was miserable every single stinking day. All I wanted to do, every day for the entire 3 weeks, was to drive to the store and down a chocolate cake. The feeling never went away and it never got easier. The cravings made me so absolutely miserable, I finally gave up and went back to bingeing.

This experience and my research led me to believe I may need to try doing my next round of hCG without the main carb/sugar sources (which on hCG are the melba/grissini and fruit), if I wanted to minimize my sugar cravings. I had never eaten the grissini, but it was quite an idea to think about removing the Phase 2 fruits entirely.

In truth, Dr. Simeon's original protocol did say that a person could eliminate anything he was not hungry for except the 2 protein servings. So there didn't seem to be any clash there.

To compensate for the pretty large calorie deficit there I decided I would add in either more P2 veggies or fat free greek yogurt that was very low in sugar, comparable in calorie content to a P2 fruit.

Was this off-protocol? Technically yes. However, Dr. Simeons did mention that occasionally fat free cottage cheese could be used in place of a protein serving, so to me, fat free greek yogurt was along the same lines, so again, in principle, this seemed like it may likely work as an alternative to my fruit.

PROBLEM & SOLUTION 5: I researched to figure out what could be causing my health symptom flare up and what I could do about it. For me this was the discovery that I was likely dealing with Adrenal Fatigue.

As I've already mentioned, the website stopthethyroidmadness.com is pretty much the best resource right now for truly up-to-date information for all things thyroid and adrenal related based on what actually works for people based on user feedback. If you are feeling very fatigued and tired, you can almost guarantee one or more hormone levels is off somewhere. I started on a physiological dose of cortisol and immediately felt much better. My energy returned and I felt happy again.

Now though, I had to consider whether continuing the cortisol dosage on hCG would negatively impact my weight loss. I knew at this point that I still needed it because I was feeling great on it, so I decided I would continue it and see how things went.

PROBLEM & SOLUTION 6: It wasn't hard to know it had been a poor choice to view being on hCG more nonchalantly that 2nd time. I felt resolved to take things seriously again. No more replacing my vegetables with sugar-alcohol cookies on hCG!

PROBLEM & SOLUTION 7: Last time, Phase 3 was a total wash because I just didn't do it. As a result I regained 15 lbs in 9 weeks. This time, I hoped that all the other changes I was implementing would leave me feeling better at the end of this Phase 2 and I would be able to enter Phase 3 feeling ready and committed.

EXPERIENCE AND OUTCOME
AFTER ADJUSTMENTS WERE MADE

OUTCOME 1: On my pre-hCG diet phase; 10 days of low carb, high fat, no sugar (including no fruit), my symptoms of sugar cravings were entirely gone after the first three days. Additionally, the symptoms I felt during those 3 days were nowhere near as acute as I had experienced previously. The way I handled it? I pretty much babied myself those first 3 days. I watched movies to distract myself. When I started thinking of ice-cream, I went and made myself up a plate of bacon. After I'd eat that, I'd feel fine again.

OUTCOME 2: Loading low carb went swimmingly well. I gained very little during the loading phase and was already in "new territory" for weight loss after the first vlcd day.

OUTCOME 3: Since my sugar cravings had dissappeared while doing my pre-hCG diet phase, and I was not eating the Phase 2 fruits or grissini, the diet did not feel hard and I continued to experience no cravings. My hunger and blood sugar felt fine eating more veggies and the greek yogurt in place of the fruit, and both my weight loss and body fat percent seemed to be going down in a very healthy way.

As a test after about 10 days on the diet, I decided to try having an apple. About a half hour after eating it, I recall sitting outside on my patio feeling a surge of sugar cravings and the desire to simply eat MORE, a lot more. I had been feeling perfectly content with my 500 calorie eating plan so far, but suddenly, it didn't feel like enough, and I as I thought about 30 more days of this, things felt bleak and very difficult to accomplish. How could I continue this diet feeling like this for another whole month? This confirmed my hunch that the sugar in fruit at that stage in getting away from my addiction to sugar and carbs, was still a problem. I didn't have any more phase 2 fruit after that, and the rest of that round felt much easier again.

OUTCOME 4: I felt very well energy-wise while using the physiological dosing of cortisol on hCG. About halfway through the round, my weight seemed to be stalling out and I had the feeling to myself that I possibly didn't need as much cortisol now. I decided to play with weaning off of it entirely over the next few days. I did this, and I continued to feel well and started losing weight again.

OUTCOME 5: When I reached Phase 3, I felt good, and stuck to P3 guidelines strictly. One thing that I ran into that was a learning experience for me is that by leaving out the fruits in Phase 2, I had depleted my glycogen stores. Glycogen is essentially sugar water that our bodies hold in our muscles and liver for quick fuel sources when needed. This meant that my final weight at the end of my round was artificially low, so I had to stabilize higher up than the 2 lb window. That was totally okay, and I was able to do hydrostatic body fat testing to show that my higher weight was due to glycogen and muscle and not fat regain. Just another example of some troubleshooting I had to do to be sure of what exactly was going on.

LONG TERM OUTCOME

I feel very good about this process, as it allowed me to stabilize and maintain. I repeated most of these steps until I got to my desired body composition, about 16-17% bodyfat. I've been hCG-free as of late 2012.

FOR YOU

This whole long narrative is to show how you can go about a thought process to troubleshoot failed attempts at this diet. Don't allow the walls you run into to stop your progress permanently. Troubleshoot!

THE 1 SECRET: Allow Time.

I used to think that as soon as a thought came into my brain, whether it was that I needed to lose weight, or that I wasn't eating healthy, that if I didn't act on it that very second, or at the very latest, tomorrow, I was a bad person somehow and I would already be a failure.

So I'd start something I wasn't prepared or ready for which of course didn't usually work out. If it did, it only ended up being a short term solution.

I had to recognize that some changes take time and that I had to synchronize my attempt at change with being mentally and emotionally ready.

That's the secret! It's *okay* if you're not ready *right now*. Wow, that was such a revelation to me.

If you gained 20 lbs in June, and you aren't mentally ready or have the best situation to do anything about it until November, that's okay.

2 Keys to This Secret of TIME

1. THE TIMING MUST BE RIGHT WHEN IT COMES TO MATCHING YOUR EFFORTS WITH YOUR MENTAL AND EMOTIONAL READINESS.

2. CHANGES THEMSELVES, ONCE BEGUN, TAKE TIME.

In fact, as I'd like to discuss, it's better to choose a time that will give you the best chance of success than to haphazardly start something.

It's kind of like this workbook. I could have put it together in a mad rush and not only would half of it be missing, it would be the half that is truly important, that may make the difference between success and failure. Some days I couldn't get any writing done on it because my brain just wasn't working. Some days I was inspired and the words just flowed. But it was worth waiting and working at it to achieve a better, much more useful resource.

After my failed round 2, I actually spent 9 weeks not being ready for hCG and not even being ready to eat healthy again. After several weeks though, I began to feel differently. I felt more open to trying again, it began to feel a little more plausible. The little workings in my brain began to tick a little more positively again. I spent the last three weeks or so of that nine

week period researching and formulating a plan for what I would do differently this next time.

By the time I was ready to begin Round 3, everything was in it's proper place and my plan worked beautifully well.

If I had not allowed myself that time, this is most likely what would have happened:

I would have tried to do hCG again immediately to "fix" what I screwed up, but the same problems would crop up and probably I would have made my situation even worse since I wasn't ready and had no plan for making the experience and outcome different yet.

ALLOW TIME, AND USE THE 2 KEYS TO THE SECRET OF TIME AS RECIPES FOR YOUR GRADUAL TRANSFORMATION.

Should a Number Be Your ULTIMATE GOAL?

200 LBS AND A SIZE 4.

OKAY THAT *could* BE AN EXAGGERATION...

I was 5'1", 128 lbs or so, a size 8, and what at the time I would call overweight, which made me depressed. That was about 10 years ago (which now, looking back, I was really not *that* overweight).

Today I'm 5'1", 127 lbs or so, a size 4, and what I would call a fit athlete (with some little pads of fat here and there just so everyone knows I'm a woman and mom hehe).

The only thing that is really different above is my clothing size.

How can I be different clothing sizes at about the same weight? How can my scale weight be the same, yet I was overweight 10 years ago and now I'm not?

It's something called body composition. Google defines composition as "the way in a which a whole or mixture is made up."

Our bodies are compositions. We focus so much on fat that sometimes we forget we're made up of some other pretty important stuff too!

The main three things that make up that number we see on the scale is muscle tissue, the water that muscle tissue holds (muscles are about 80% water), organ, bones, fat, and more water.

None of us are trying to lose bones or muscle right? We all agree this is the stuff we want to keep,

or even improve in some way yes? Fat takes up more space on our bodies by weight than our other components (aside from looking more....blobby, than bones and muscle look).

YOU COULD BE 200 LBS BUT IF YOU WERE A SIZE 4, WOULD YOU COMPLAIN? Now obviously, I'm exaggerating a bit here, but just to make this point. I think ultimately what we care about, or what makes sense to care about, is our physical size and shape, not our weight.

HCG AND EXERCISE TO REFINE THE INGREDIENT RATIOS OF YOUR BODY

You can ***refine*** the composition of your body with this protocol. You can ***change*** how much of you is fat and how much of you is muscle, over time, through the use of the hCG protocol and working out (specifically lifting weights) ***in between your rounds of hCG***, which is what I did to achieve my current body. This means you ***may*** end up being a higher weight than you originally thought you needed to reach. This is a good thing!

Muscle doesn't just take up less space than fat on your body, making you slimmer at a higher weight, it also helps you maintain a healthier metabolism so that you can have a higher calorie intake without gaining weight. Also a very good thing!

Here's the other weird thing about the ***look*** of fat vs. muscle. Muscle does still take up space on your

Happiness and Health AS AN ULTIMATE GOAL.

body right? If I weigh 110 lbs with 90 lbs of me being muscle and 20 lbs of me fat, or I weighed 125 lbs with 105 lbs of me being muscle and 20 lbs of me fat, **even though I have the same amount of fat in both cases**, I'm still going to physically be a little bigger at 125 lbs vs. 110 lbs because the extra muscle still takes up space.

HOWEVER, BEING PHYSICALLY BIGGER DUE TO MUSCLE RATHER THAN DUE TO EXCESS FAT LOOKS A LOT DIFFERENT.

Your body will have a much smoother appearance to it so that you *still* look small and fantastic, even if you are one size up in your favorite jeans. I'm not kidding here! This may be hard to believe, but it's true.

HOW TOO-SPECIFIC
SCALE WEIGHT GOALS
CAN BACKFIRE

Being focused solely on a specific number on the scale can be counterproductive if you want to get fit and experience greater ease in maintaining by having a higher ratio of muscle on your frame. Muscle does weigh something! If you want to improve your muscle mass after losing fat with hCG, this will mean that you will have some added "weight."

But this doesn't mean your physical size has to be large. I'm practically in the red zone when it comes to my scale weight according to weight charts you find online for my height. However, because so much more of me is muscle and so much less of me is fat than the average person of my height, my body fat percent shows that I'm actually in the athlete category, and I wear a size 4

to prove it.

TRY TO BE STUCK *less on scale numbers* AND

MORE ON THE CLOTHING SIZE
THAT MAKES YOU FEEL MOST COMFORTABLE IN YOUR OWN SKIN.

. . . .

2 STARTING VIEWPOINTS
HOW EACH CAN EFFECT YOUR PROGRESS.

There are 2 opposite viewpoints that I've seen us ladies coming from when we begin this protocol and I'd like to talk about how each can your weight loss and weight maintenance efforts.

The first way you can look at it, which I think is a good starting place is this:

THE *"At this point I'll be happy to be just a little overweight instead of a lot overweight!"* MENTALITY.

This is how I was thinking of it when I began hCG. I had gotten so overweight for my height, at 172 lbs and had become so hopeless, that **I felt just being able to get into a size that I previously had considered overweight still would be quite acceptable to me and I'd be happy with that.** In high school I was a size 2, but at a size 16/18 at my highest I thought if I could just get to a size 8 again, I'd be happy! I didn't need to look like a model anymore, I just wanted to be smaller than I was then.

After my first round and seeing how effective the protocol was, *I started to realize getting leaner was actually within my grasp in a reasonable way. This made me modify my goals.*

In retrospect, I feel this was a healthy way to look at it because it allowed me to be happy on a continual basis with my progess. I didn't have to reach some pie-in-the-sky goal to feel a sense of accomplishment. Each pound shed, each size drop, made me feel elated. These were just the sort of positive feelings I needed to experience to keep driving me forward on the journey.

As I said, seeing how feasible weight loss was on this particular protocol, I was able to modify my goals to get leaner than I originally intended, while still reaping the benefits of keeping my expectations low overall so that I could feel happy during my entire journey instead of only at the end.

This road isn't a short one. Even though hCG weight loss can be quick, once you factor in all the phases and the breaks and the difficult transitions mentally and emotionally, it ends up taking up a lot of time actually. You don't want to have to wait till the very end of it all to feel a sense of pride in yourself. You want to be able to feel good about yourself the entire journey.

This attitude also helped me in maintaining my weight, because once again, I learned to have a more reasonable outlook on my body. I learned to have a spectrum that I feel my body looks good at. For me that's about a 7 lb range. I look fantastic at 127 lbs and I look even more fantastic at 120 lbs. Even though I do maintain a pretty small size these days, I no longer have a fat-detection honing device on my person, noticing every pad of fat and hating it. What I see is a woman of reasonable size, and I am happy with this.

The 2nd way we sometimes approach the hCG

protocol that can pose a problem is this:

THE "I'm so glad I found hCG, now I can be 5'10" and 120 lbs" MENTALITY.

Sometimes we discover the hCG diet and immediately create a very specific, **"ultimate"** goal weight right away, which is usually pretty much the absolute best physique our genetics would allow if we were still 18 years old. Sometimes having such a lofty goal, especially right away, can backfire a little bit.

One drawback to having a goal that is both too specific and too advanced at the very start is that you may miss out on feeling good about yourself during the journey. When you hit rough patches, your end point will start to seem so far away that it can cause excessive discouragement.

Additionally, some ultimate goals that are grand in nature, may not lead to ultimate happiness.

When deciding what you will be happy with, what your "ultimate goal" will be, ask yourself these 2 questions:

What weight can I maintain relatively easily and be a reasonable size? At what weight can I still have a life?

If you reach the thinnest weight you can possibly reach without being downright unhealthy, but to maintain this weight you must count every calorie, portion every item that goes in your mouth, never have a night off, and pretty much live and breathe your daily diet in order to stay that weight, is it worth it?

If you have long range reasons for weight loss, like family, living longer, health, etc., living a life consumed by diet would take you in the opposite direction of your goal.

How can we be satisfied with our bodies in a balanced way?

What is reasonable when it comes to our bodies?

To me, it's *a weight you can maintain in a do-able, still-live-my-life sort of way, and be a reasonable size.*

This doesn't mean that I haven't made some drastic changes to the way I eat on a daily basis. I have. I don't insist that I still be able to eat fast food daily and maintain or I give up.

But you will find that there is a balance between the main healthful eating habits that you will establish, and a way of life that you are able to live *happily*, that equates to what sort of body you can maintain.

I am pretty fit. Am I as thin as I was in high school? No. I don't live and breathe food restriction like I did back then. Sure I was a size 0 but I was also miserable and paranoid much of the time.

Do I panic if I miss crossfit 1 day out of the week? Nope. Do I panic if I eat fries one night? Nope. I have an 80/20 type lifetsyle, and this allows me to have what I guess you could call 80% of the absolute best physique possible for my genetics. For me, this is the happy balance for how I want to *live* my life. To reach the 100% level for my body would mean a life lived in a way that couldn't actually be enjoyed, so that's not worth it to me.

Finding your happy balance, the level of change and dedication you are willing to put into your future daily life for maintaining a certain type of body may be different.

WOA, WHAT??

Woa, looks like I've officially gone off my rocker. Why in the world would anyone recommend your goals be vague?

Well, for all the reasons that we just discussed, but let's recap.

The reason in this case that making your bigger, more long-range goals vague in nature, is that you may not likely know just yet what is the best final outcome for your body.

Making specific goals prematurely can cause discouragement or may cause you to pursue something that isn't actually in your best interests.

Having a more general goal at the beginning; losing weight and getting into smaller clothing, and then re-assessing at various points, will give you the freedom to make and pursue more specific goals when the times comes that are more appropriate, both for happiness and health.

Remember, you can always modify your weight loss goals as you go along. You are not locked into anything!

What I encourage you to do, though, is to:

KEEP HAPPINESS AND HEALTH AS YOUR MAIN DRIVING FACTORS WHEN MAKING GOALS.

KEEPING BIG GOALS VAGUE

Never Say Never...OR SAY NEVER...

To be perfectly honest, I had no intention of changing my eating habits for the long haul when I initially came across the hCG protocol. I didn't see any realistic way to change, given how addicted to sugar and food I was.

One very valuable secret I have learned through this process though is that:

YOUR STATE OF BEING TRULY DOES CHANGE AS YOU GO THROUGH THIS JOURNEY.

The result of this? What feels impossible today, will feel quite do-able, even easy, in a couple months.

This is because the many minor adjustments you will be making as you go through the hCG diet will change you.

But living in a very different way, i.e. eating a much altered daily diet compared to your prior way of eating, in order to maintain weight loss, will not be attainable if you don't actually begin the journey.

CLARITY AND CAPABILITY COME WITH APPRENTICESHIP

Clarity, or you being able to *see* how you will be able to live in a new way, comes as you apprentice that new way of life and become capable as a result.

What do I mean?

Imagine an apprentice to a trade. What allows an apprentice to move on a full-fledged expert, not just in name but in actual ability as well? The skills they learn during that time as an apprentice right?

For a very skilled position, it seems likely that a brand new apprentice who knows nothing about the field might be at a total loss if presented with a bunch of high level tasks they haven't been trained to do yet. Not only would they feel completely overwhelmed, they probably wouldn't be able to carry them out, at that point.

But the long term solution in this case is that the very act of apprenticing will teach the person the skills needed to carry out such tasks very capably. So the obvious choice is **not to project fear over the future** assignments that are as yet not undertsood, but to use the time apprenticing to learn.

You are putting trust in yourself that you will be able to learn and you will **then** be capable. You base your feelings and actions for the future **on** the future and what you plan on doing in the mean-time leading up to that.

This same thing happens when making lifestyle changes.

What you don't feel capable of doing now, you will be learning how to do as you go through this, and you will be capable at the end.

Some aspects of the learning process may feel tougher to learn than others, but it will be happening in a gradual, progessive manner.

This means that what you can't comprehend being capable of doing now, you will feel confident of being able to handle later.

That is how my own weight loss journey unfolded. While I couldn't fathom giving up sugar or complete freedom with carbs for good, I figured I could somehow manage to stay on a diet for 40 days if I was going to lose a lot of weight doing it. I figured I'd deal with what I was going to do afterwards....afterwards!

BUT THEN **EMBARK** ON THE JOURNEY ANYWAY.

I had no idea what I was in for. No clue the metamorphosis I would undergo. The losing weight portion of the diet; eating 500 calories, was certainly no snuggly fireside evening, but I did manage to get through it and what is most interesting is how I felt when I began Phase 3.

Prior to beginning the hCG protocol, no exaggeration, I had a daily compulsion to get either a quart or half gallon of ice-cream, or a large package of cookies, or several donuts. I couldn't go an entire day without one of these items. It was truly a daily "fix" I had to have, or I would be very distracted with obsessive thoughts about it, wondering when/where/how I could get one of these things before bedtime without my family noticing.

After completing Phase 2 of the hCG protocol, it had now been a full 6 weeks since I'd eaten anything unhealthy or binged on something sugary. Instead I had been consuming only whole foods, and the very small amount of sugar I had consumed had only been in whole fruit form.

My first morning of Phase 3, I barbecued up a grass fed burger patty, a large bowl of veggies that I roasted on the grill, and shared a Phase 3 friendly smoothie (just water, frozen blueberries, ice and stevia) with my mom. And it was *divine*. Truly satisfying in every way. I didn't sit there wishing it were donuts or cookies or ice-cream.

And it felt like that again the next day. And the next. Just reveling in my new Phase 3 eating lifestyle - clean, whole foods, no sugar. It not only felt easy, it felt like what I actually *wanted*.

So, if you are feeling scared or overwhelmed about how you are going to make long term changes based on how you feel right *now*, remember this:

YOUR STATE OF BEING TRULY DOES CHANGE AS YOU GO THROUGH THIS JOURNEY.

The result of this is that what feels impossible today, will feel quite do-able, even easy, in a couple months.

Plan your HCG ROUND AHEAD for best results

Sometimes you have a vacation coming up. Sometimes there are 6 social engagements planned during a 3 week period. These are typically not the best times to be on a round of hCG- you'll know why as soon as you try to do it. It's just hard. Planning ahead and finding a low key period in your life to do a round of hCG will really help you be successful.

MONTH: YEAR:

MONTH: YEAR:

MONTH: **YEAR:**

MONTH: **YEAR:**

Section

2

· · · ·

DIET
INSTRUCTIONS

5 Steps - hCG Diet BASICS

STEP #
1
START TAKING HCG. LOAD FOR 2 DAYS ON HIGH FAT/HIGH CALORIE FOODS.

STEP #
2
PHASE 2 3-6 WEEKS. TAKE HCG WHILE ON THE 500 CALORIE DIET.

STEP #
3
TRANSITION OFF HCG. 72 HOURS.

STEP #
4
PHASE 3. 3 WEEKS. NO HCG. STABILIZE.

STEP #
5
PHASE 4. LIFE. GRADUALLY ADD STARCHES BACK IN.

Take hCG. PHASE 1: LOADING PHASE

You begin taking hCG the morning you start the "Loading Phase" where you spend 2 days eating high fat/high calorie foods. Many often gain weight during this 2 day period, but it comes off quickly when you begin the diet portion.

A. WHAT TO EAT. You can eat whatever you like, however, the emphasis should be on high fat items. If you want more ideas go to hcgchica.com/loading

Take hCG. PHASE 2: 500 CALORIE DIET

Time to lose weight folks. The 500 calorie diet portion or VLCD (very low calorie diet) is typically referred to as Phase 2 (P2) and lasts 3-6 weeks to complete 1 "round" of the hCG diet. **You will follow the rules for the 500 calorie diet. The food list is very specific, as is how the food is portioned out.**

No hCG. TRANSITION: GET OFF HCG

About 72 hours is needed for hCG to get out of your system, during which time your body will still be more sensitive than usual to fats and calories. To transition off it, stop hCG but continue the 500 calorie diet for 72 hours following your final dose of hCG.

No hCG. PHASE 3: STABILIZE WEIGHT

Time to stabilize your new weight. This involves eating no sugars or starches for 3 weeks following Phase 2. During this time you will be attempting to keep your weight within 2 lbs of your LDW (Last Dose Weight - your weight on the scale the morning of your last hCG dose). If your weight goes more than 2 lbs above your LDW:

A. *a* STEAK DAY: Eat nothing for the main part of the day, drink lots of water. For dinner: Eat a large steak and tomato or apple.

No hCG- PHASE 4: EAT & MAINTAIN

Gradually try adding back in healthy starches and sugars. Ideally certain foods you won't be returning as a habit if they weren't somewhat healthy, but at this point you can experiment with healthy carbs and occasional treats. Some choose to just live a Phase 3 eating lifestyle. Others find they can maintain their weight eating some carbs but not others. It will be a bit of experiment discovering what your body is okay with. Just to encourage you, I have been able to maintain while eating a normal amount of healthy carbs since 2012.

PHASE 1 *loading*

Dr. Simeons' original protocol involves eating:

A HIGH FAT, HIGH CALORIE DIET FOR AT LEAST 2 DAYS, WHILE TAKING HCG AT THE SAME TIME.

This is just prior to beginning the low calorie diet.

In his words, the patients were to "eat to capacity of the most fattening food they can get down until they have had their third injection."

Most load for 2 days. Dr. Simeons suggested that those who had been doing a lot of chronic dieting just before starting this protocol load for more days, so if this is you, 1-2 extra days may be considered.

He suggested highly concentrated foods such as, "milk chocolate, pastries with whipped cream, sugar, fried meats particularly pork, eggs and bacon, mayonnaise, bread with thick butter and jam, etc."

So essentially, you *can* eat whatever you like during this time period with the focus on foods high in fat, however, you may want to see my note below under loading modifications.

Usually there is some weight gain during the loading phase, but on occasion a person actually loses. Either result is perfectly fine.

In general, most people (including myself) lose all the loading weight within 2 days on the 500 calorie diet.

Just to give you an example of how many calories you may end up consuming, on my final round of hCG I ate 4000 calories and about 300 grams of fat *each* loading day. You will most likely feel pretty full. However, I don't personally think it's necessary to make yourself sick during this process as that just doesn't seem sane or healthy to me. Be balanced.

NOT ORIGINAL PROTOCOL

PHASE 1 *loading Modifications*

Without going into too many details, I found through trial and error that when **doing this loading phase without the use of sugars and starches I fared better in a few ways.**

1. Bingeing on sugar and carbs as some do with traditional loading was too much like my previous binge eating disorder, something I was trying to get away from.

2. Some will get into Ketosis during Phase 2 (a state where fat reserves are tapped into much more easily, from what I gather) and loading without carbs allows you to get into this state much faster.

3. Cravings during the first week of the low calorie diet are usually less and hunger goes away more quickly.

4. Detox symptoms like experiencing cravings and feeling flu-ish during first week of Phase 2 are usually minimized.

To do this, I ate lots of meat and low carb vegetables slathered in butter and oil, as well nuts, seeds and some dairy products like full fat sour cream and cheese.

This is simply an option, not mandatory. I have used this method with good success as the end result.

You can get all my latest content related to the loading phase at hcgchica.com/loading

hCG Injection DOSAGE

Dr. Simeons originally dosed his patients with hCG at 125IU by injection, once a day. Today there are many weight loss clinics dosing patients with a wide range of dosages.

The following is just my observation based on feedback from several hundred people and my own personal experience (and remember I'm not a medical professional).

It appears that *the dose of hCG one takes has a direct bearing on the feeling of hunger or non-hunger during this diet, and what this best dosage is, is unique to you* - even from round to round this number can change. Additionally, it's surprising how very small dosage changes can take you from feeling half starved to experiencing an almost complete lack of hunger.

I can tell you, if there is one thing that will physically make you feel the urge to quit on this protocol, it's excessive hunger for days on end.

I encourage you to coordinate with your doctor on these two following areas so you can have the best experience on hCG, both with weight loss and hunger:

2 THINGS YOU MAY WANT TO RESEARCH FURTHER

1. Dialing in the best dose for you personally for minimal hunger.

2. How to gauge when an adjustment in dose may be in order and whether you need a higher or lower dose.

You may find the following detailed article helpful to address these two factors in the most effective way, based on what has worked for myself and many others:

hcgchica.com/dosage

hCG Diet TIMELINE

HOW LONG SHOULD YOU STAY ON THE HCG DIET?

This is not your typical diet where you start it and then stay on it until you're done losing weight. Instead, this diet is done in what are called "rounds". You do the diet for 3-6 weeks at time. Then you take a break and stabilize your new weight. Then you start a new round of hCG to lose additional weight. You repeat this until you are where you want to be.

The original window of time Dr. Simeons designated to do a round of hCG just had 2 rules:

> DO AT LEAST 23 INJECTIONS
>
> DON'T GO BEYOND 40 INJECTIONS WORTH (including loading day injections)

THE BASIC IDEA I GET OUT OF THAT IS TO DO THE DIET FOR 3-6 WEEKS OR SO.

In general, if you have a larger chunk of weight to lose, it makes logistical sense to do longer six week rounds. When you don't have as much to lose, motivation is often not as high and in these cases, the three week rounds are often more fitting.

In the end, rather than committing yourself to one length of time in advance, see how you feel as you go. Some start out desiring to do a full six week round only to discover that they are feeling really burned out by week four. I've had multiple people report to me that they handle doing shorter, more numerous rounds much better mentally and emotionally.

You always want to give a high level of respect to your emotional and mental capacity to handle this protocol. Once that becomes too compromised, you're in the danger zone for cheating and re-gaining weight.

It's better to stop when you are feeling that super "done" feeling. This is not the same feeling as when the diet sometimes feels very difficult at the beginning, or when you have an occasional tough day. I'm talking about when you're halfway or three quarters of the way through a round, and you are starting to have a constant "I'm so done and I don't care anymore" type of feeling that keeps sticking with you multiple days in a row.

HOW LONG SHOULD YOUR BREAK FROM THE HCG DIET BE?

Here are the designated breaks that Dr. Simeons outlined in his original protocol:

BETWEEN ROUNDS:	BREAK:
1 AND 2	6 WEEKS
2 AND 3	8 WEEKS
3 AND 4	10 WEEKS
4 AND 5	12 WEEKS
5 AND 6	14 WEEKS

As you can see two additional weeks off is added to each subsequent round, so you keep adding if you do more rounds than this.

To see what you DO during these breaks, check out the Phase 3 and Phase 4 guidance on pages 70-73.

CHANGING IT UP

Some wonder if these breaks are necessary, or if they can do rounds longer than 6 weeks or shorter than 3 weeks. For more detailed discussions on these ideas, go to *hcgchica.com/timing*

PHASE 2 PRINCIPLES - *Losing Weight*

GOAL FOR PHASE 2:

Allow the hCG hormone to interact with your body to both change your sensation of hunger, as well as protect your lean muscle tissue, while your body taps into your abnormal fat reserves to fuel your daily living, thereby allowing quicker fat loss than is usually possible.

STEP # 1 ## CALORIES ARE KEPT VERY LOW.

STEP # 2 ## CARBS ARE A SMALL AMOUNT.

STEP # 3 ## AVOID INGESTION OF FATS AND OILS IN ANY FORM.
(thru skin or mouth, except mineral oil)

These are the 3 basic principles that the rules of the hCG protocol are based on that seem to correlate with proper weight loss while the hCG hormone is in your system. When considering whether or not to make a modification to the diet, keeping these 3 principles in mind will help you make wise choices.

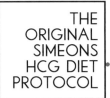
PHASE 2 RULES *the 500 Calorie Diet*

Non-protocol foods that some now use are shown in grey boxes.

Approved FOOD LIST

Remove all visible fat
Do not cook with skin

PROTEINS:

Meat serving size:
100 grams/3.5 ounces

- Lean Beef
- Chicken breast
- Veal
- Fresh white fish

Types of White Fish

Catfish
Cod
Flounder
Halibut
Sole
Red Snapper
Sea Bass
Tilapia
Trout

- Lobster
- Crab
- Shrimp

Occasional Meat Replacement:
- 1 egg + 3 egg whites
- 100 grams fat free Cottage Cheese

Off-Protocol PROTEINS
- 99% Fat Free Ham
- Turkey Breast
- Tuna (Water Packed)
- Protein Shake (low carb)

VEGETABLES:

There is no serving size for veggies listed in the original protocol.

- Asparagus
- Beet Greens
- Cabbage
- Celery
- Chard
- Chicory
- Cucumber
- Fennel
- Lettuce
- Onions
- Radishes
- Spinach
- Tomatoes

Off-Protocol VEGGIES
- Bell Pepper
- Broccoli
- Mushrooms
- Yellow Squash
- Zucchini

FRUITS:

- 1 Apple
- ½ Grapefruit
- 1 Orange
- Strawberries *(handful)*

Off-Protocol FRUITS
- Blackberries *(handful)*
- Blueberries *(handful)*
- Raspberries *(handful)*

CARB:

- 1 Grissini Stick
  (Not allowed if these contain olive oil- check ingredients.)
- 1 Melba Toast

SMALL STUFF:

- Juice of 1 lemon/day
- 1 tablespoon milk/day
- Stevia* or saccharin
- Salt, spices, herbs, vinegar etc. ok as long as they don't contain sugar, starch, or oil.

Off-Protocol OTHER
- Miracle Noodles
- Fat Free Greek Yogurt
  (in place of fruits)

*Stevia was not included in the original protocol, since it was written in the 50's before Stevia was even around in most countries. It is a standardly accepted sweetner on this protocol however, and in this day and age, considered to be a healthier option than saccharin.

Please note: I don't necessarily endorse all modifications to the diet. It's your personal choice whether you include them in your Phase 2. To see what modifications I personally used, and under what circumstances I used them, see pages 62-67, or go to: hcgchica.com/modifications

THE CALORIES
How to Portion

ALL FOOD CHOICES SHOULD BE COMING FROM THE APPROVED FOOD LIST.

BREAKFAST:
Coffee or tea

LUNCH:
- 1 protein
- 1 vegetable
- 1 fruit
- 1 carb

DINNER:
Same as lunch.

Additional INSTRUCTIONS *at a glance*

More details/explanations on these additional instructions in the next pages!

DO'S:
» Drink 2 liters (about 2 quarts) of liquid a day.
» The 100 grams of meat must be weighed raw.
» Remove all visible fat from the meat. Meat should be as lean as humanly possible. 80/20 ground beef won't do.
» Skip one injection a week if doing the diet >3 weeks (continue diet as normal).
» Skip hCG but continue the diet during menstruation.

CANS:
» You can break up the 2 meals as much you like, making multiple snacks out of a meal if you choose, ie. take a fruit from lunch and eat it for breakfast, etc.
» Sugar free items can be used tentatively. Don't go overboard.
» You can eliminate anything you are not hungry for **except** the protein servings.

» If weight loss stalls for a few days in a row, an Apple Day may be done.
» Treatment interruptions are allowed if necessary by taking a short break of less than 2 weeks during Phase 2.

CANT'S:
» Do not use makeup or skincare products containing oil unless it's mineral oil.
» Avoid any skin contact with oil (except mineral oil).
» Do not combine multiple servings into one meal- ie. eating two fruit servings at once, or two proteins at once.
» There's no restriction on the size of a single apple, but you can't eat two small apples in place of one large.
» Do not mix vegetables at a meal.
» Massages are not allowed.

ORIGINAL DIET:
DO'S

		HCGCHICA SIDE NOTES:

DRINK 2 LITERS OF LIQUIDS A DAY.

Toxins are stored in fat, so drinking enough water while on hCG is wise as it will help your body flush out toxins that may get into your bloodstream as your body metabolizes your fat for fuel.

WEIGH THE 100 GRAMS OF PROTEIN RAW.

When weighing meat that's already been cooked, you will want to aim for a portion size less than 100 grams as raw meat contains a higher water content. A good rule of thumb would be 70-80 grams per serving of cooked meat.

REMOVE ALL VISIBLE FAT FROM MEAT.

hCG makes your body a lot more sensitive to fats. It's important for any meat you eat to be as lean as humanly possible. So 80/20 ground beef won't work.

SKIP 1 INJECTION A WEEK IF DOING THE DIET >3 WEEKS (CONTINUE DIET AS NORMAL).

It doesn't hurt to do this, so you may as well. This was insituted by Dr. Simeons as a way to prevent immunity that he said occurred in some patients. I haven't actually seen this happen in practice for some reason. You don't have to panic if you didn't skip a shot for a few weeks. Just do it as a precaution when you remember.

SKIP HCG BUT CONTINUE THE DIET DURING MENSTRUATION.

I chose to skip hCG on my heaviest flow days only - for me this was 1-2 days. From my observation it is a good idea to do this because otherwise sometimes hCG can cause issues with menstruation, either preventing it entirely or causing it to last longer than normal, while on hCG.

ORIGINAL DIET:
CAN'S

YOU CAN BREAK UP THE 2 MEALS AS MUCH AS YOU LIKE.

What this means is that you can make multiple snacks out of a meal. Examples: Take the lunch fruit serving and have it for breakfast. Or weigh 50 grams of protein and save the other 50 grams for lunch. Saving a dinner fruit for late night snack.

YOU CAN ELIMINATE ANYTHING YOU ARE NOT HUNGRY FOR EXCEPT THE PROTEIN SERVINGS.

This means there may be times you are actually eating less than 500 calories. This is okay IF you are truly not hungry. Hunger is largely hCG dose dependent. If you are experiencing excessive hunger on hCG, you likely need an adjusted dose.

SUGAR FREE ITEMS CAN BE **TENTATIVELY** USED.

Tentatively means hesitantly or experimentally. Many find Stevia to be fine, some use Splenda. But in some cases if you are on the leaner side you may be more ed by sugar free sweeteners, or if you are using too much of them. Sugar alcohols are more iffy - use them sparingly as too much does indeed blood sugar which will weight loss on hCG. My personal opinion is Splenda is unhealthy - google that one.

ORIGINAL DIET:

HCGCHICA SIDE NOTES:

IF WEIGHT LOSS **STALLS** FOR A FEW DAYS IN A ROW, AN APPLE DAY CAN BE DONE.

Apple days involve eating *up to* 6 Apples, minimizing water intake, and eating nothing else. Apple days begin at noon one day and end at noon the following day. Keep in mind Dr. Simeons mentioned the main objectives of doing this were to help you emotionally while dealing with the stall, and to get rid of excess water retention. Doing an apple day involves eating a lot more carbs than usual and no protein, so keep that in mind when deciding to do one or not.

TREATMENT INTERRUPTIONS TAKING A SHORT BREAK FROM HCG DURING PHASE 2.

If something comes up and you need to be off hCG and the diet for 2 weeks or less, you can do an interruption. Technically only to be done after you've already used 23 injections worth otherwise weight regain during the break is more likely. This involves getting off hCG as if you were finishing Phase 2, with the same 72 hour transition period (see page 68 for instructions). Eat Phase 3 style to hunger (calories may end up being somewhere between 800-1600). When ready to resume hCG no re-loading is necessary, simply start hCG and the very low calorie diet again to finish out your round.

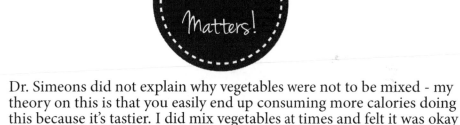

ORIGINAL DIET:

CAN'T'S

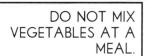

DO NOT MIX VEGETABLES AT A MEAL.

Dr. Simeons did not explain why vegetables were not to be mixed - my theory on this is that you easily end up consuming more calories doing this because it's tastier. I did mix vegetables at times and felt it was okay for me. If you DO choose to mix some P2 vegetables together, be more conscious of how *much* you are eating.

DO NOT COMBINE MULTIPLE SERVINGS INTO ONE MEAL

Examples: Do not eat both fruit servings at once, or the two protein servings for the day at the same time.

AVOID ANY CONTACT WITH OILS ON THE SKIN.

The hCG hormone makes your body more sensitive to fats than usual - both to losing it and gaining it. Our skin is our largest organ. Let me repeat that. Our skin is our largest organ. I am inclined to believe Dr. Simeons that fats and oils on our skin will cause problems during the diet. Wear gloves when cooking with fat.

DO NOT USE MAKEUP OR SKINCARE PRODUCTS CONTAINING OILS BESIDES MINERAL OIL.

Same argument as above. I have a free ebook download on hcgchica.com/makeup called *"Mac to Maybelline - Makeup and Skincare Products Safe to Use on the hCG Diet"* that was researched by a skincare specialist who checked ingredients for oils in common brands.

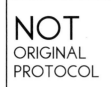
PHASE 1 - LOADING *Modifications*

> These are a couple of modified methods I utilized that encompass just prior to the loading phase of hCG, and the loading phase (P1) itself.

1 WEEK PRE-HCG DIET

If you begin this diet with fairly healthy eating habits, you probably won't need this measure.

However, that wasn't me. I started the hCG diet addicted to sugar. I had developed a binge eating disorder of sorts where I ate large amounts of sugary foods on a daily basis. If you have sugar or carb addict tendencies, you may find this method helpful!

My sugar cravings and withdrawal symptoms were pretty intense during the first couple weeks on the hCG protocol. **This literally brought me to the very brink of giving up** entirely on my first round. I was in despair at the thought relinquishing my only hope for change.

I did some research into how I could better prepare myself for future rounds so that I could avoid such intense sugar/carb withdrawals during hCG. What if there was a better, less intense way of getting off sugar *before* the hCG diet began?

I found that a 7-10 day "pre-hCG diet" if you will, of eating a low carb/high fat diet achieved this for me. It's important that I iterate the importance of not simply eating low carb but **high fat** as well. I utilized this for my final 3 rounds and it worked - wonderfully.

To do this I ate only higher fat protein, low carb veggies, and had a carefree hand with fats like butter, olive oil, cheese, avocados, and nuts. I removed most carbs, even fruit. During the first few days, every time I had a major hankering for ice-cream or some such nonsense, I cooked myself up a plate of bacon. This method really did accomplish the two things I desired.

1. It made the sugar cravings go away permanently so it was not a daily battle.

2. It shortened the withdrawal symptom time frame to a few days and made it less severe while it lasted.

I'm not endorsing a long term diet of mass bacon consumption folks! This was a short term means to an end. If you are vegan, choose high fat foods that don't contain many carbs.

One thing I should mention about this. If you do this little Pre-hCG Diet thing, your overall weight loss on your actual round of hCG might seem lower than average from loading to the end of Phase 2.

This is because you may lose the water weight you would usually lose with hCG, *before* hCG. That's what any type of low carb eating does.

Don't let this throw you off, just know what is happening so you don't have to be worried that your results are not as good.

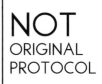
You might choose to keep track of your weight during this time period as a reference for your total weight loss, and I have created a quick glance tracking chart just for this should you choose to utilize this.

Now, if you do the Pre-hCG Diet, and then do the 2 day loading phase with sugar and carbs, you will likely have a larger looking gain on the scale as your body recovers it's glycogen stores that may have been depleted during the low carb period of the Pre-hCG phase, but this will also likely come off very quickly as soon as you start the low calorie diet since it is mostly water weight.

If you load clean, without sugars and carbs, which is discussed next, you will most likely have a very minimal loading gain.

CLEAN LOADING:
LOADING PHASE WITHOUT SUGAR OR CARBS.

Some of the examples Dr. Simeons gave for typical loading foods during Phase 1 were things like milk chocolate and baked goods.

I found my sugar/carb cravings and the ease of sticking to the diet were much better when I loaded on high fat foods but completely eliminated all sources of sugar and regular carbs (including fruit) during the loading phase.

CLEAN LOADING FOODS INCLUDE:

» Higher fat meat, bacon, or lean meat with liberal butter or other fat.

» Low carb veggies, with lots of butter/coconut oil/olive oil.

» High fat items like avocados and olives.

» Low carb homemade breads made with flax and chia type stuff slathered with lots of...you guessed it, butter.

» Dairy: Cheese, full fat yogurt, sour cream, heavy whipping cream (higher fat dairy items have fewer carbs).

» Low carb smoothies made with protein powder, a lavish amount of coconut milk or avocado, water or almond milk (sugar free kind), ice cubes and stevia.

» Nuts: These have more carbs than you might think, so make them an element of clean loading vs. the main ingredient.

» Small amounts of sugar free sweeteners like stevia and erythritol.

WHAT TO AVOID COMPLETELY:

» Common carbs ie. grain, pasta, beans, etc.

» Anything containing any form of sugar - ie. brown/white sugar, brown rice syrup, agave syrup, honey, etc.

» Fruit

» Higher Carb Veggies ie. potatoes, beets, cooked carrots, peas, etc.

So rather than cake and pie, it was more a 2 day fest on bacon, steak, and butter type deal. The main difference between the 7-10 pre-hCG diet phase and the clean loading? Clean loading involves a higher calorie intake with the main purpose being fat intake. I was not so concerned about veggie intake and such during loading.

PHASE 2 *Modifications*

The following foods are not part of the original Simeons protocol. These are items that I personally incorporated into my own hCG journey at various points as described below, and I feel comfortable enough with the results that I would use these same variations again.

Additionally, the way I did Phase 2 itself at various points was a little different, and again, I feel the results for me were good, so that's why I've chosen to include them as options for you to consider.

Whether you choose to modify the foods on the diet is up to you. One practical way to go about it is to start out completely POP (perfect on protocol) and then gradually, as you become bored out of your mind or feel like you're about to cheat, use those points in your journey to try a slight modification, instead of just quitting or cheating. It will help keep the protocol fresh and make it feel less like it's taking forever.

Remember that making modifications in an informed and judicious manner is not the same the thing as cheating on the diet. ***If you make irresponsible choices on this protocol, you will be affected negatively by it. That is not what I'm endorsing here.***

ADDITIONAL FOODS *I ate during Phase 2*

PROTEINS:

» Ground Turkey - 99% fat free
» Canned Water Packed Tuna
» 97% fat free Ham

VEGETABLES:

» Bell pepper - any color
» Zucchini
» Yellow Crooked Neck Squash
» Mushrooms
» *Small* bits of raw carrot

OTHER:

» 0% Fat Free Greek Yogurt
» Miracle Noodles / Shirataki Noodles / Zero Calorie Noodles
» Stevia/erythritol sweetened sodas. *(very occasional)*
Brand ideas: Blue Skye and Zevia

PHASE 2 *Modifications*

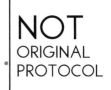

Notes on OFF PROTOCOL VEGETABLES

I would use 1/4 or 1/2 of a bell pepper in salads. For mushrooms, I'd take one whole package, slice them and then simmer them in water for my soup base, add a few herbs and my 100 grams of chicken breast or shrimp with salt to taste. Repeat but with zucchini or crookneck squash for other meals. I would often add Miracle Noodles to these bowls of soup. The small bits of carrot? I would literally shave a quarter of a raw carrot into a P2 salad. Just enough to give the salad some taste and texture.

Notes on OFF PROTOCOL PROTEINS

While I did use canned tuna on occasion and know a number of others with great results who did as well, my feeling is that it's something to be cautious with as mercury pollutant levels are fairly high in tuna. I feel this may be a concern while you're trying to lose weight. Toxins may be stored in fat so I feel it could present a problem for your body trying to process toxins from fat loss while new ones are coming in from unsafe food sources. Regarding ground turkey, it's 99% fat free - this is something that I don't think was common or accessible when Dr. Simeons created his protocol in the 1950's. The main principle to follow when choosing a meat protein source are 1. as close to fat free as possible, and 2. avoiding meats that contain too many hormones. The ham I would slice up small and make a chopped salad with.

Notes on OFF PROTOCOL "OTHER STUFF"

FAT FREE GREEK YOGURT

I have used this both in place of my Phase 2 fruits and to make my own "ranch" dressings for my salads. As a replacement for my P2 fruit, I would have a 60 calorie serving (for the brand I bought that amounted to about 1/2 cup) and added a little stevia to make it sweet. As a dressing, I would use just a teaspoon or so, with a dash of vinegar and salt, on my P2 salad, and it was DELISH!

MIRACLE NOODLES / SHIRATAKI NOODLES / ZERO CALORIE NOODLES

These noodles are calorie free - they are purely soluble fiber. I used them, either as a half package or even a whole package, per Phase 2 meal, on a daily basis for 3 of my rounds, mostly in soups. Keep in mind that percieved "weight gains" from using these noodles are due to water retention and additional bulk in your intestines, which will go away. I do not believe it has anything to do with your actual fat loss on the diet. To see my full explanation and review go here: *hcgchica.com/noodles*

STEVIA AND ERYTHRITOL SWEETENED SODAS

These are something **I would use only on occasion**, for instance a social gathering, so I felt less desperate while the stuffed mushrooms were being passed around. I don't recommend their use on a regular basis while on Phase 2. In tiny amounts I don't see the erythritol being an issue, but in large amounts it seems that it can affect blood sugar, which could then interfere with fat loss during this phase. Depending on how lean you are getting, even small amounts may be an issue, so pay attention and be willing to take things out when you're not sure.

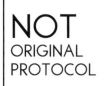
PHASE 2 *Modifications*

MIXING VEGETABLES.

Even though Dr. Simeons instructed not to mix vegetables during Phase 2, I did so on a round and feel this worked out fine for me.

The key here is, if you do this, you need to be more conscious of the *amount* of veggies you are eating, as once you start combining them, everything starts getting tastier and you can overshoot portions more easily.

Additionally, **on the round that I mixed vegetables I was not eating P2 fruit.** I replaced those calories with more P2 vegetables (discussed next), so I felt this gave me more leeway when it came to the vegetables on the diet.

To give you an example of the way that I mixed vegetables, I would for instance have a salad of lettuce, half a cucumber, and 1/4 piece of carrot shaved very thin *(note: carrot is off protocol - use at your own risk)* just for flavor.

NO FRUIT:
REPLACE WITH FAT FREE GREEK YOGURT.

I did not do this on every round. I utilized this for 2 rounds as a way to eliminate cravings from my sugar addiction. Other rounds when I was feeling more in control of my eating in general, I was able to include P2 fruit as part of the diet without issues.

Dr. Simeons actually did state you could eliminate any food you weren't hungry for on the diet, except the 2 protein servings. So that part is not off protocol.

However, on 2 of my hCG rounds, I chose to *replace* the calories from the P2 fruit servings with 60 calorie portions of fat free greek yogurt. You should compare brands when choosing and use the one with the lowest sugar content, as they do vary greatly. I added a little stevia to my yogurt so it was more of a sweet snack.

Again, this method worked well for me when I was inititally breaking my sugar addiction, as at that time I found even healthy fruit would trigger sugar cravings.

MIRACLE NOODLES.

A brand name for a type of noodle also packaged as Shirataki noodles, these are calorie free and have zero net carbs. How is that possible??

They're made of a water-soluble fiber from the root of an asian plant called the Konjac.

You can see a video review of me showing and discussing them in more detail, as well as where to purchase them at:

hcgchica.com/noodles

PHASE 2 *Modifications*

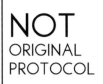

What I like about these noodles is that they create a feeling of satiety very easily because of their volume. Add them to Phase 2 soup recipes for a very satisfying meal.

One thing to keep in mind: because of their bulk as well as the water that the fiber noodles will absorb, after you first introduce them to your diet you may notice either no weight loss or even a gain the following day.

I used these noodles almost daily on three of my rounds, and I do not feel they hampered my actual fat loss. Any gains or zero loss days appeared to be tied to the bulk of the noodles themselves and the water they absorbed while in my intestines.

THE 5 MODIFICATIONS
TO THE HCG DIET:

That's it. The five main modifications I employed at various points in my hCG weight loss journey. Remember that I did not utilize all these modifications for every round, and each one was done under specific circumstances and for specific reasons.

1. ONE WEEK PRE-HCG DIET

2. CLEAN LOADING – PHASE 1

3. MIXED VEGETABLES – PHASE 2

4. NO FRUITS – PHASE 2

5. MIRACLE NOODLES – PHASE 2

Fixing a DIET CHEAT

Cheating on this protocol is one of those things you want to avoid like poison oak. It just ain't pretty. You won't die, but it can lead to inordinate gains and take days to recover from.

Yet sometimes it just happens doesn't it? What then? Is it all over? Is everything ruined? Should you just head over to your local donut shop to drown your sorrows inside a pink box with a baker's dozen?

Actually there *is* something you can do to get yourself back on track, so please don't feel overly discouraged. This is simply a small gopher hole you stepped in on your trail to success.

This is the method I used to recover from a cheat more quickly:

> **ELIMINATE PHASE 2 FRUIT**
> the following day or two and
> **EAT MORE**
> **PHASE 2 VEGETABLES**
> **INSTEAD.**

This is a way to clear excess carbs from your system more speedily and get your body back to losing fat.

If you are already not eating Phase 2 fruit on the diet anyway, or you just feel really bummed that you screwed up, remind yourself of this:

IT ALREADY HAPPENED.
Will feeling so bummed that you give up help?

It's in the past now. Let it go, and move on. This mistake will only prevent you from succeeding if you allow the cheat to your decisions going forward. If you move on, chin up, everything will be alright.

For more detailed help on recovering from cheats and how to avoid them in the future, please go to
hcgchica.com/cheating

TRANSITION OFF HCG *72 hours till P3*

About 72 hours is needed for your body to process the last of your hCG dosing, during which time it will still be more sensitive than usual to fats and calories. To transition off it, Dr. Simeons original instructions were to **stop hCG but continue the very low calorie diet for 72 hours following your final dose of hCG.**

WHEN DOES THE 72 HOUR PERIOD BEGIN AND END?

The 72 hour transition period begins immediately following your final dose of hCG. The minute you inject yourself for the last time or take your last set of drops, the 72 hour race to your first Phase 3 smoothie recipe you got off Pinterest is *on*.

Handy Dandy WHEN DOES P3 START CHART

THOSE TAKING INJECTIONS:

Example: If your last dose is at 9 am, P3 will start at 9 am on the day designated on the chart.

THOSE USING DROPS/PELLETS:

Example: If your last dose of hCG is at 7pm, P3 will start at 7pm on the appropriate day.

Last hCG Dose:	1st Day of Phase 3:
SUNDAY	WEDNESDAY
MONDAY	THURSDAY
TUESDAY	FRIDAY
WEDNESDAY	SATURDAY
THURSDAY	SUNDAY
FRIDAY	MONDAY
SATURDAY	TUESDAY

I'm going to tell you my experience. Towards the end of the 72 hours - the last 24 hours or so, I had discovered myself not only feeling very hungry, but getting symptoms of low blood sugar. Since the hCG hormone level *is* gradually reducing in your body during that 72 hours, it stands to reason that you might get hungrier as that 72 hours unfolds.

As such, you may find the need to gradually increase your calories, still from the Phase 2 food list, as the 72 hours wears on *if* you find yourself getting very hungry. The need to do this will vary from person to person - leaner people will most likely be a lot more aware of hunger as the 72 hours is finishing. I feel it's not a good idea to force yourself to stick to the 500 calories at this point if hunger really does become an issue, because it can backfire and cause overeating and lack of control during the first few days of Phase 3, something you really want to avoid.

My guesstimate on additional calories you may find yourself needing during the last 24-48 hours is 200-500 calories.

SHOULD YOU INCREASE CALORIES AS THE 72 HOURS GOES BY?

HOW TO DO IT

- » Be vigilant about keeping fats/oils out of the picture still.
- » Eat more Phase 2 foods *as necessary* (based on your hunger), likely in the 200-500 calorie range.
- » Best choices are probably additional meat protein and/or vegetables.

PHASE 3 RULES *- Stabilizing Your New Weight*

GOAL FOR PHASE 3:

Stabilize your new weight. It takes about 3 weeks of eating in the manner described below for your weight to go from being volatile, to stable. According to Dr. Simeons, you are a creating a new set point.

STEP # 1
NO STARCHES OR SUGARS FOR 3 WEEKS FOLLOWING PHASE 2.

Essentially a low carb diet.

STEP # 2
KEEP YOUR WEIGHT WITHIN 2 LBS OF YOUR LDW.

Your LDW (last dose weight) is your weight recorded the morning of your last dose of hCG.

STEP # 3
IF YOUR WEIGHT GOES ABOVE 2 LBS, DO A STEAK DAY.

A steak day is eating nothing until dinner, drinking lots of water throughout the day, then having a large steak with apple or tomato for dinner.

NOTE! I highly encourage you to get a lot more details on successfully navigating Phase 3 either through: *hcgchica.com/p3* or you can follow my fully-structured phase 3 program at *p3tolife.com*

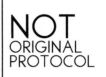

TIP #1: If You Want To Be EXTRA CAUTIOUS

You don't *have* to do these things, but if you want to be extra cautious, or are having trouble stabilizing your weight with the basic rules, these four additional measures can really help:

A. EAT TO HUNGER. ie. eat to be satisfied but not overly full.

B. INTRODUCE CALORIES/AMOUNTS OF FOOD GRADUALLY.

C. INTRODUCE DAIRY AND NUTS SLOWLY, OR WAIT TILL PHASE 4 to add one or more of these food groups. These are common food sensitivities. You may notice a gain when you eat something you are allergic or sensitive to, and adding these foods slowly helps you keep track of these weight gain triggers.

D. INTRODUCE FATS CONSISTENTLY BUT RAISE THE AMOUNT SLOWLY. I wouldn't wait until Phase 4 to add fat back in, but you might not want to start day one of P3 with six slices of bacon either. I find people seem to stabilize better and also feel best when it comes to digestion when they incorporate a small amount of fat at the beginning, and gradually raise this amount over the three week period.

TIP #2: If You Have to Do Steak Days STAY IN P3 LONGER.

If your phase 3 has been so rocky that you've done several steak days, it's likely that by the end of the three weeks your weight is still not very stable.

Ideally you want to spend a good few weeks really having a fairly stable weight before attempting to incorporate too many higher carb items again.

The idea is that your body is ready to handle carbs once it's *been* stable for a bit.

TIP #3: Remember the POINT OF P3

There are times when you may choose to stabilize at a higher weight than the 2 lbs. THE POINT OF THIS PHASE IS TO BECOME STABLE AT A NEW LOWER WEIGHT.

Whether it's 2 lbs, or 4 lbs higher, in the end doesn't really matter. You might stabilize UNDER 2 lbs. Try to not to get too focused on a specific number so much as the goal of seeing your weight become steady.

TIP #4: Eat REAL FOOD

It's possible that before this diet you had some less than healthy eating habits. I did. Make this a time to continue the eating of REAL WHOLE FOODS with as little processing as possible.

I've been surprised at how much a difference additives, chemicals, and the like, while being "calorie free", can make in our efforts to both stabilize and maintain weight.

TIP #5: Get More DETAILED INFO

I have a some free p3 guidance on my blog hcgchica.com/p3 as well as a fully structured Phase 3 program at **p3tolife.com** to help you through this phase. P3 is just not as reliable or easy to navigate as Phase 2. My phase 3 to life program actually makes it a piece of cake to navigate & you will see many video interviews of ladies testifying to this at **p3tolife.com/interviews**.

There are a bunch of "special case" scenarios, depending on how you chose to do Phase 2 of the diet, that will affect where and how to effectively stabilize in P3.

Space just doesn't all me to discuss all this here, so please do go to p3tolife.com to learn more.

GOAL FOR PHASE 4:

FIND YOUR NEW NORMAL: HOW YOU WILL BE ABLE TO EAT IN REGULAR LIFE, SEPARATE FROM THE HCG PROTOCOL, WHILE STILL MAINTAINING YOUR WEIGHT LOSS. DISCOVER WHAT CARBS YOUR BODY HANDLES WELL, AND WHICH ONES IT DOESN'T.

Phase 4 is what many call the maintenance phase, meaning it's pretty much the way you want to be eating in regular day to day life once you are done losing weight, while still maintaining your weight loss, which ideally will include some carbs.

However, when you begin Phase 4 the idea is to **adapt** your body to carbs again, as well as **discover** what carbs your body tolerates well and which ones it doesn't.

The best way to do this is to add carbs back in gradually, both in quantity and type.

Tracking the carbs you incorporate back into your diet on a trial basis allows you to be more aware of what action may be causing a certain result, so you are better able to make the needed adjustments to keep your new body in balance. You can do this with the coming companion Phase 3 & 4 hCG Diet workbook. *Find more info on this at hcghica.com/workbooks*

Your Phase 4, your healthy, normal, way-of-life-eating, will no doubt morph and adapt as time goes on. I've been in phase 4 since late 2012 and I've adjusted how and what I eat several times. My current favorite snack that doesn't cause me to gain weight is peanuts. Several months before this it was toasted organic corn tortillas with butter. In the coming companion Phase 3 & 4 workbook, I go into detail on the 3 factors that help create your personal Phase 4 lifestyle.

PHASE 4 = YOUR NEW NORMAL

P4 is not static. It's about trying out new foods, in a gradual manner, to achieve your new typical way of eating, derived from a marriage of 3 things:

» the **health factor**
» the **"what makes the scale go up"** factor
» the **sanity factor**

The health factor, the "what makes the scale go up factor" and the sanity factor.

This will help you to look at things in a balanced way and find ways to respect your body's possible negative reaction to some foods while still feeling freedom and not deprivation in your life.

I've discovered it's truly how you feel mentally more than the actual freedom or restriction that allows you to feel content, happy, and to continue with a certain way of eating.

TIPS FOR GETTING STARTED IN PHASE 4

1. Add one new carb at a time. ie. potato, *or* rice, not both at the same time.

2. Add quantities of carbs gradually.

3. Note bodily reactions to these changes. These can include weight gain, puffiness, feeling swollen, digestive troubles, etc.

4. Temporarily remove foods your body seems to react badly to, and try again at a later time to see if the same thing happens.

5. Keep records of foods to avoid and foods that seem to be fine so you know what you *can* eat.

As hCGer Nance said once,

WHEN YOU FINISH PHASE 2, YOUR WEIGHT IS LIKE WET CEMENT.

IT CAN GO TWO WAYS IN PHASE 3. YOU CAN PAY NO ATTENTION TO WHERE YOU'RE GOING AND STOMP AROUND ON IT AND MESS IT UP GRANDLY, OR YOU CAN TREAT IT PROPERLY AND CAUTIOUSLY AND IT WILL CURE AND SOLIDIFY IN ITS PLACE.

There is no truer statement than this in the hCG world. I have seen so many ladies **work so hard in P2 only to have it all come back afterwards,** simply because **they didn't know exactly what to do to stabilize** and maintain their new weight loss. This led to what my 2 year project creating:

the PHASE 3 to LIFE PROGRAM

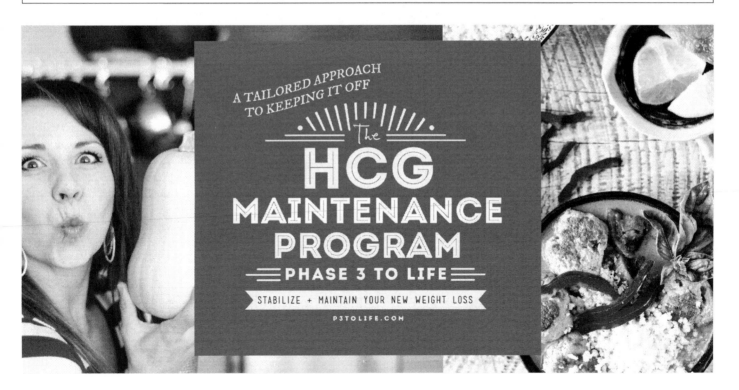

When I initially released this fully structured Phase 3 to life program ("to life" as in helps lead you into maintaining weight loss long term as well), I was literally overcome-crying-head-in-my-hands freaking out over whether this would actually help you ladies stabilize and maintain. Just because you spend a lot of time and research creating something, doesn't mean it will work for sure. I went ahead and released it despite the crazies I felt in my head, and all those feelings are now gone. You know why? Because it works.

Once you ladies took the program for a test drive the results were even better than I could have hoped to hear. Lady after lady needed no correction days, stabilized, in some cases lost weight, didn't feel hungry and said they felt like they were cheating because the food was so good and filling.

You can hear it from their mouths on video here:

P3TOLIFE.COM

Section

3

. . . .

QUICK GLANCE
PROGRESS

Starting **PHOTO**

DATE: _____   CLOTHING SIZE:

WEIGHT: _____   pants: _____

ROUND #: ____   shirts: _____

Ending **PHOTO**

DATE: _____   CLOTHING SIZE:

WEIGHT: _____   pants: _____

LBS LOST: ____   shirts: _____

Psst! Over here! **I'D LOVE TO SEE YOUR HCG PROGRESS.** If you'd like to share your results so far, email me your story and photos to **hcgchica@hcgchica.com. I read all your stories personally.** To check out other real hCG success stories, go to **hcgchica.com/interviews**

Tracking INCH LOSS

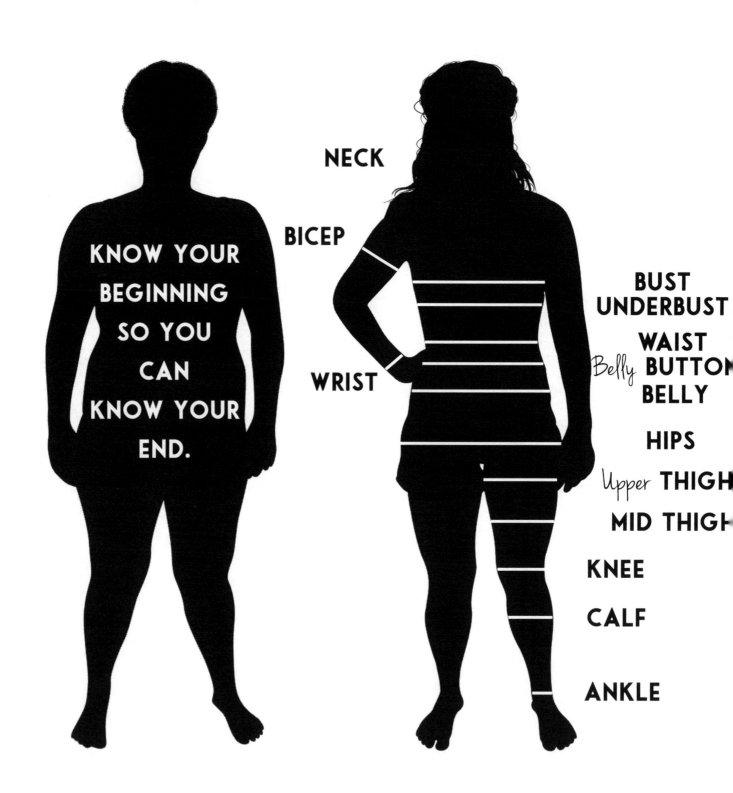

KNOW YOUR BEGINNING SO YOU CAN KNOW YOUR END.

NECK

BICEP

WRIST

BUST
UNDERBUST
WAIST
Belly BUTTON
BELLY

HIPS

Upper THIGH

MID THIGH

KNEE

CALF

ANKLE

Finding the RIGHT SPOT

Neck — Huh? Yeah, I never would have thought to measure this either, except I saw a gal on youtube do it. I lost **1 INCH** off my neck in my 50 lb weight loss, and of my hCG interview guests (Episode 18) lost **4 INCHES** from her neck in her 110 lb weight loss. So wrap that tape around your neck.

Bicep — Measure the widest part of the middle of your arm- if you slide the measuring tape up and down your arm by a couple inches you should be able to find this spot.

Wrist — Another one of those places that you might not think to measure! Most of us, if we get overweight enough, get little pads of fat on our wrists. These do indeed go away as you lose weight.

Bust — Measure the widest part of your chest - usually right across the nipple line.

Under Bust — **Under-what?** I had never heard of this term before, but this is an excellent place to measure because most of us have those infamous bra-area rolls there- by measuring directly under your breast area you will get to see this area shrinking. Just to be clear, the area you will measure is DIRECTLY under your breasts- so if you have a larger bust, the measuring tape will essentially be underneath them.

Waist Area — There are varying opinions on where your waist really is. I find the following the easiest way to be consistent about where I'm measuring:

WAIST: Measure the tiniest part of your trunk. That could be a few inches above your belly button.

BELLY BUTTON AREA: Measure directly across the area of your trunk where your belly button is.

BELLY: Measure the widest part of your middle. Yes the hanging belly fat area.

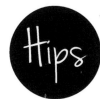

Hips — You want to measure around the widest part of you in this area.

Legs — Being consistent in these areas can be tricky. You may not get it perfect everytime.

UPPER THIGH: Measure the widest area of your upper thigh- where it bulges the most. Usually this will be just below the crease of your buttocks.

MID THIGH: I found this spot to be one of the trickiest when it comes to measuring the same spot consistently. You want to shoot for halfway between your knee and the very top of your thigh.

KNEE: Measure the widest part across your knee.

CALF: Measure the widest portion of your lower leg. Usually this is several inches below your knee.

ANKLE: Again, you want to find the widest circumference of your ankle area and measure there. For most this will probably be just above your ankle bone.

Tips on MEASURING YOURSELF

① Measure once a week or less.

Don't measure yourself too frequently you guys. There's a couple reasons for this:

For one, the whole point of measuring is to encourage you. You won't likely see much difference from one day to the next and this could end up making you feel discouraged instead.

The second reason is just one saltier-than-usual meal, or a hot day (you know when your fingers get all puffy?) can temporarily increase certain measurements. This has nothing to do with fat gain. It can be all too easy to start over-scrutinizing and driving yourself crazy.

By sticking to once a week you'll likely see inches go down on various parts of your body which will be rewarding.

Even then, measuring every week could be too much. Remember, **the key is whatever you're doing should help you feel motivated and encouraged. If you find it's doing the opposite, skip it!**

② Measure in the morning.

Try to measure under the same conditions. Ideally I find it best to do when you first wake up in the morning, after a pee run, and before you start drinking and eating which can throw off the measurements.

③ Myotape tape measure

This little tool called the **Myotape Body Tape Measure** tool makes it much easier to get accurate and consistent measurements. Easy to find online and inexpensive at about $5.

④ Stick with the right or left side.

For your limbs, choose one side to measure, either right or left, and stick with it.

I was surprised to discover my legs are not the same! One is consistently about 3/4" thicker than my other. If I had switched back and forth without realizing it, my tracking would have been off and I could have gotten discouraged.

Remember, even though you're only measuring one arm and one leg, the inch loss is happening on both sides! Include this when you're counting up your inch loss.

If you have extra time or are rather anal, ahem, detailed oriented like me, you might end up deciding to just measure both sides of yourself all along.

Tips on MEASURING YOURSELF

5

Measure Friday vs. Monday.

Cheating happens most often on weekends because that's when people usually find themselves in compromising situations during social occasions.

While you don't want to plan to cheat, you might figure that Friday mornings might be an ideal time to measure yourself, when you've had almost a whole week of sticking well to the protocol.

This just might also be a little added encouragement to help you stay strong through whatever difficulties the weekend presents when you see the progress you are making.

6

Don't panic over inch increases.

Sometimes we experience the B word, bloating, around our menstrual cycles, ovulation, due to dehydration, or when we have more salt than usual (did you have soup last night?)

If you notice what seems like an inch increase, or no decrease, when measuring your trunk area, no need to spaz, likely one of the above reasons is the culprit.

7

Not too tight or too loose.

I think the tendency is to err on the side of pulling the tape too tight; could be a subconscious desire to see those inches go down as fast as possible!

But really, you want to try to use a consistent hand when using the tape measure. You don't want it tight enough that it's cutting into the flesh that you are measuring, but also not so loose that the tape is sagging on part of you.

It should lie flat against your skin. The myo tape I referred to in tip #3 I find is pretty nice for this.

8

Don't hold your breath.

I realized that when I would measure my belly I would tend to kind of suck my breath in. Don't.

Later if you don't suck your breath in you'll freak out that you've "gained" an inch. :)

My INCH LOSS RESULTS

"It had long since come to my attention that people of accomplishment rarely sat back and let things happen to them. They went out and happened to things."

–LEONARDO DA VINCI

ROUND # ☑1 ☐2 ☐3 ☐4 ☐5 ☐6 ☐7 OTHER: ____

Starting MEASUREMENTS

VLCD 0	DATE 9-4	A.M. WEIGHT	165.9	
NECK	13"	HIPS	42	
BICEP	LT= 13" RT= 10"	UPPER THIGH	L 24	R 24 1/2
WRIST	Lt- 7" Rt - 6'12	MID THIGH	L	R
BUST	39	KNEE	L	R
UNDER BUST		CALF	L 15 1/2	R 15 1/2
Smallest part of WAIST	36" RL 6'12	ANKLE	L 10	R 10
BELLY BUTTON	37	OTHER		
BELLY		OTHER		

End OF ROUND Last Dose Weight Measurements

VLCD DAY:____	DATE	A.M. WEIGHT		
NECK		HIPS		
BICEP		UPPER THIGH	L	R
WRIST		MID THIGH	L	R
BUST		KNEE	L	R
UNDER BUST		CALF	L	R
Smallest part of WAIST		ANKLE	L	R
BELLY BUTTON		OTHER		
BELLY		OTHER		

My INCH LOSS

Location	DATE 9-4 VLCD# WEIGHT 165.4	DATE VLCD# WEIGHT 159.2	DATE VLCD# WEIGHT	DATE VLCD# WEIGHT	DATE VLCD# WEIGHT	DATE VLCD# WEIGHT	DATE VLCD# WEIGHT	DATE VLCD# WEIGHT	INCH LOSS TOTALS
NECK	13	13							
BICEP	LT-13" RT-13"	13'							
WRIST	Lt 7" Rt 6½	13'							
BUST	39"	38½							
Under BUST		33							
WAIST	35"	33	33						
Belly BUTTON	37"	35	35						
BELLY									
HIPS	42"	40	40						
Mid THIGH	L R	L R	L R	L R	L R	L R	L R	L R	
Upper THIGH	L 24 R 24½	L 24 R 23½	L R	L R	L R	L R	L R	L R	
KNEE	L R	L 17 R 17	L R	L R	L R	L R	L R	L R	
CALF	L R	L 15½ R 15	L R	L R	L R	L R	L R	L R	
ANKLE	L 10" R 10"	L 10 R 10	L R	L R	L R	L R	L R	L R	
OTHER:									
OTHER:									

Tracking INCHES AFTER HCG

Location	DATE WEIGHT	DATE WEIGHT	DATE WEIGHT	DATE WEIGHT	DATE WEIGHT	DATE WEIGHT	DATE WEIGHT	DATE WEIGHT
NECK								
BICEP								
WRIST								
BUST								
Under BUST								
WAIST								
Belly BUTTON								
BELLY								
HIPS								
Mid THIGH	L R	L R	L R	L R	L R	L R	L R	L R
Upper THIGH	L R	L R	L R	L R	L R	L R	L R	L R
KNEE	L R	L R	L R	L R	L R	L R	L R	L R
CALF	L R	L R	L R	L R	L R	L R	L R	L R
ANKLE	L R	L R	L R	L R	L R	L R	L R	L R
OTHER:								
OTHER:								

The 7-10 day Pre-hCG Diet, as discussed in more detail in the Modifications to hCG section, is an **optional** method I found useful for addressing sugar addiction in the quickest, most effective, and least painful manner possible. If sugar/carb addiction is not something you struggle with, this may not be an important thing for you to do.

If you **do** choose to implement this tactic, you **may** lose a little weight, but you may not. Either result is perfectly normal.

DATE	TIME	DAY	WEIGHT	+ OR –	TOTAL LOSS	NOTES
		7–10 DAY PRE-HCG DIET				
		DAY 1				
		DAY 2				
		DAY 3				
		DAY 4				
		DAY 5				
		DAY 6				
		DAY 7				
		DAY 8				
		DAY 9				
		DAY 10				

WEIGHT TRACKING CHART- **PHASE 2**

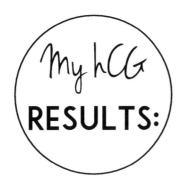

My hCG **RESULTS:**

FINAL RESULTS		
TOTAL LOADING GAIN:	7	
STARTING WEIGHT:	162.9	**LDW** (last dose weight):
WEIGHT LOSS – GROSS:		
WEIGHT LOSS – NET:		

Let's get this show on the road!

Please note! I chose to label the first day of the low calorie diet as day 0 for the following reason: Weight loss doesn't start adding up until *after* the first vlcd day. The morning of the eighth day on the diet, your written entry will show how much you've lost after seven full days, one full week, on the 500 calorie diet.

DATE	TIME	DAY	WEIGHT	+ OR –	TOTAL LOSS	NOTES	INJEC-TION #
9-4	9:00	LOAD DAY 1	162.9		– WEEK 1 –		
9-5		LOAD DAY 2	165.2				
9-6		LOAD DAY 3 (if applicable)	169.00				
9-7		VLCD 0					
9-8		VLCD 1	164.8				
9-10		VLCD 2	160.8				
9-11		VLCD 3	161.4				
9-12		VLCD 4	159.2				
9.13		VLCD 5	159.2				
		VLCD 6					
		VLCD 7	160.2			Take Measurements Day	

WEEK **1** WEIGHT LOSS TOTAL:

Remember! There is often a good portion of weight loss at the start of any diet that is water weight loss - this will often lead to an epic looking first week. The weight loss will naturally decrease in general once the excess water weight is gone. This is normal and expected. The ensuing weeks will be accomplishing a lot of fat loss for you which will greatly change your body, even if the "pounds" lost seem like less than the first week.

WEIGHT TRACKING CHART- PHASE 2

DATE	TIME	DAY	WEIGHT	+ OR –	TOTAL LOSS	NOTES	INJECTION #
WEEK 1 ENDING WEIGHT:				– WEEK 2 –			
		VLCD 8					
		VLCD 9					
		VLCD 10					
		VLCD 11					
		VLCD 12					
		VLCD 13					
		VLCD 14				Take Measurements Day	

WEEK 2 WEIGHT LOSS TOTAL:

DATE	TIME	DAY	WEIGHT	+ OR –	TOTAL LOSS	NOTES	INJECTION #
WEEK 2 ENDING WEIGHT:				– WEEK 3 –			
		VLCD 15					
		VLCD 16					
		VLCD 17					
		VLCD 18					
		VLCD 19					
		VLCD 20					
		VLCD 21				Take Measurements Day	

WEEK 3 WEIGHT LOSS TOTAL:

DATE	TIME	DAY	WEIGHT	+ OR –	TOTAL LOSS	NOTES	INJECTION #
WEEK 3 ENDING WEIGHT:				– WEEK 4 –			
		VLCD 22					
		VLCD 23					
		VLCD 24					
		VLCD 25					
		VLCD 26					
		VLCD 27					
		VLCD 28				*Take Measurements Day*	
WEEK 4 WEIGHT LOSS TOTAL:							

DATE	TIME	DAY	WEIGHT	+ OR –	TOTAL LOSS	NOTES	INJECTION #
WEEK 4 ENDING WEIGHT:				– WEEK 5 –			
		VLCD 29					
		VLCD 30					
		VLCD 31					
		VLCD 32					
		VLCD 33					
		VLCD 34					
		VLCD 35				*Take Measurements Day*	
WEEK 5 WEIGHT LOSS TOTAL:							

Quick Glance
WEIGHT TRACKING CHART- PHASE 2

DATE	TIME	DAY	WEIGHT	+ OR –	TOTAL LOSS	NOTES	INJECTION #
WEEK 5 ENDING WEIGHT:				– WEEK 6 –			
		VLCD 36					
		VLCD 37					
		VLCD 38					
		VLCD 39					
		VLCD 40					
		VLCD 41					
		VLCD 42				Take Measurements Day	

WEEK 6 WEIGHT LOSS TOTAL:

DATE	TIME	DAY	WEIGHT	+ OR –	TOTAL LOSS	NOTES	INJECTION #
WEEK 6 ENDING WEIGHT:				– WEEK 7 –			
		VLCD 43					
		VLCD 44					
		VLCD 45					
		VLCD 46					
		VLCD 47					
		VLCD 48					
		VLCD 49				Take Measurements Day	

WEEK 7 WEIGHT LOSS TOTAL:

WEIGHT TRACKING CHART- PHASE 2

DATE	TIME	DAY	WEIGHT	+ OR –	TOTAL LOSS	NOTES	INJECTION #
WEEK 7 ENDING WEIGHT:				– WEEK 8 –			
		VLCD **50**					
		VLCD **51**					
		VLCD **52**					
		VLCD **53**					
		VLCD **54**					
		VLCD **55**					
		VLCD **56**				*Take Measurements Day*	
WEEK **8** WEIGHT LOSS TOTAL:							

DATE	TIME	DAY	WEIGHT	+ OR –	TOTAL LOSS	NOTES	INJECTION #
WEEK 8 ENDING WEIGHT:				– WEEK 9 –			
		VLCD **57**					
		VLCD **58**					
		VLCD **59**					
		VLCD **60**					
		VLCD **61**					
		VLCD **62**					
		VLCD **63**				*Take Measurements Day*	
WEEK **9** WEIGHT LOSS TOTAL:							

Quick Glance WEIGHT TRACKING CHART- **PHASE 3**

Check out my structured Phase 3 program at *p3tolife.com*

DATE	TIME	DAY	WEIGHT	+ OR –	NOTES
		P3 DAY 1			
		P3 DAY 2			
		P3 DAY 3			
		P3 DAY 4			
		P3 DAY 5			
		P3 DAY 6			
		P3 DAY 7			
		P3 DAY 8			
		P3 DAY 9			
		P3 DAY 10			
		P3 DAY 11			
		P3 DAY 12			
		P3 DAY 13			
		P3 DAY 14			
		P3 DAY 15			
		P3 DAY 16			
		P3 DAY 17			
		P3 DAY 18			
		P3 DAY 19			
		P3 DAY 20			
		P3 DAY 21			

TROUBLESHOOTING *log*

Even though the majority of your experience on the hCG protocol is just the natural way that things go, and I definitely don't encourage over-analyzing, there are times when there may be a legitimate *thang* going on that may be inhibiting you in some way. This is a place to consider possible reasons for trouble you may be having. It could be dealing with constipation, trouble sleeping, weight loss issues, possible food intolerances, not drinking enough water, etc. Most importantly, this will help you give thought to what adjustments you can try out to remedy the problem.

DATE: _____

VLCD #: _____

Possible PROBLEM: _____

Possible Causes	Adjustments to Try	Results

DATE: _____

VLCD #: _____

Possible PROBLEM: _____

Possible Causes	Adjustments to Try	Results

DATE: _____
VLCD #: _____

Possible **PROBLEM:**

Possible Causes	Adjustments to Try	Results

• • • • • • • • • • • • • • • • • •

DATE: _____
VLCD #: _____

Possible **PROBLEM:**

Possible Causes	Adjustments to Try	Results

• • • • • • • • • • • • • • • • • •

DATE: _____
VLCD #: _____

Possible **PROBLEM:**

Possible Causes	Adjustments to Try	Results

• • • • • • • • • • • • • • • • • •

DATE: _____

VLCD #: _____

Possible
PROBLEM:

Possible Causes	Adjustments to Try	Results

• • • • • • • • • • • • • • •

DATE: _____

VLCD #: _____

Possible
PROBLEM:

Possible Causes	Adjustments to Try	Results

• • • • • • • • • • • • • • •

DATE: _____

VLCD #: _____

Possible
PROBLEM:

Possible Causes	Adjustments to Try	Results

• • • • • • • • • • • • • • •

DATE: _____
VLCD #: _____

Possible PROBLEM: _____

Possible Causes	Adjustments to Try	Results

• • • • • • • • • • • • • • • •

DATE: _____
VLCD #: _____

Possible PROBLEM: _____

Possible Causes	Adjustments to Try	Results

• • • • • • • • • • • • • • • •

DATE: _____
VLCD #: _____

Possible PROBLEM: _____

Possible Causes	Adjustments to Try	Results

• • • • • • • • • • • • • • • •

Section

4

. . . .

DAILY
TRACKING
AREA

SOME DAYS WILL CERTAINLY FEEL *hard*.

BUT TRY TO REMEMBER THAT MOST OF THE TIME

THOSE FEELINGS **WILL** *pass* AND THE ENSUING DAYS

WILL BE MORE DOABLE.

Week 1

"DREAMS ARE RENEWABLE.
No matter what age or condition, there are still untapped possibilities within us and new beauty waiting to be born."

- Dr. Dale Turner

Please note! Most only do the loading phase for two days. The third day is optional/not usually necessary.

LIFE BEGINS AT THE END OF YOUR COMFORT ZONE.

A flower does not think of competing with the flower next to it - **IT JUST BLOOMS.**

LOAD DAY 1 (Date): _____

WEIGHT: _____

HCG DOSAGE: _____

TOTAL CALORIES: _____

SUPPLEMENTS: _____

☐ Multivitamin ☐ B12 Shot ☐ Lipo Shot

LOADING FOODS/MEALS EATEN

LOAD DAY 2 (Date): _____

WEIGHT: _____

HCG DOSAGE: _____

TOTAL CALORIES: _____

SUPPLEMENTS: _____

☐ Multivitamin   ☐ B12 Shot   ☐ Lipo Shot

LOADING FOODS/MEALS EATEN

LOAD DAY 3 (Date): _____

WEIGHT: _____

HCG DOSAGE: _____

TOTAL CALORIES: _____

SUPPLEMENTS: _____

☐ Multivitamin   ☐ B12 Shot   ☐ Lipo Shot

LOADING FOODS/MEALS EATEN

VLCD 0 (Date): _____

WEIGHT: _____

HCG DOSAGE: _____

HUNGER LEVEL: _____

BEDTIME/WAKE TIME: _____

HOURS SLEEP: _____

TOTAL CALORIES: _____

SUPPLEMENTS: _____

☐ Multivitamin ☐ B12 Shot ☐ Lipo Shot

HCGCHICA TIP:
Don't underestimate the power of sleep in both the quantity and quality (fat vs. muscle) of your weight loss.

INJECTION LOCATION   TIME: _____

☐ Belly ☐ Deltoid ☐ Thigh ☐ Other: _____

DROPS / PELLETS DOSE TIMING

1st Dose: _____   2nd Dose: _____
3rd Dose: _____   4th Dose: _____

PERSONAL NOTES

....

....

....

....

....

....

....

....

LIQUIDS:

4 LITERS	128 oz = 1 GALLON
3.5 LITERS	120 oz
3 LITERS	112 oz
2.5 LITERS	104 oz
2 LITERS	96 oz = 3 QUARTS
1.5 LITERS	88 oz
1 LITER	80 oz
.5 LITERS	72 oz
	64 oz = 2 QUARTS
	56 oz
	48 oz
	40 oz
	32 oz = 1 QUART
	24 oz
	16 oz
	8 oz = 1 CUP

BREAKFAST   Time :

☐ None ☐ Fruit: _____   ☐ Protein: _____   Calories: _____

Serving Size: _____   Serving Size: _____

LUNCH Time :   WAS AN ITEM EATEN AS A SNACK? WHICH?   Time:

Protein:
- ☐ Chicken breast
- ☐ Beef
- ☐ Veal
- ☐ Shrimp
- ☐ Lobster
- ☐ White fish: _____
- ☐ Protein Shake
- ☐ Other: _____

Serving Size:
- ☐ 100 grams/3.5 oz
- ☐ Other: _____

Calories: _____

Vegetable:
- ☐ Asparagus
- ☐ Beet Greens
- ☐ Cabbage
- ☐ Celery
- ☐ Chard
- ☐ Cucumber
- ☐ Fennel
- ☐ Lettuce
- ☐ Onions
- ☐ Radishes
- ☐ Spinach
- ☐ Tomatoes
- ☐ Other: _____
- ☐ Other: _____
- ☐ Other: _____

Calories: _____

Fruit:
- ☐ Strawberries
- ☐ ½ Grapefruit
- ☐ Apple
- ☐ Orange
- ☐ Other: _____

Starch:
- ☐ Grissini
- ☐ Melba
- ☐ Other: _____

Calories: _____

Other:
- ☐ TBS. Milk
- ☐ Juice of 1 Lemon
- ☐ Stevia
- ☐ Shirataki/Miracle Noodles
- ☐ Other: _____
- ☐ Other: _____
- ☐ Other: _____

Calories: _____

DINNER Time :   WAS AN ITEM EATEN AS A SNACK? WHICH?   Time:

Protein:
- ☐ Chicken
- ☐ Beef
- ☐ Veal
- ☐ Shrimp
- ☐ Lobster
- ☐ White fish: _____
- ☐ Protein Shake
- ☐ Other: _____

Serving Size:
- ☐ 100 grams
- ☐ Other: _____

Calories: _____

Vegetable:
- ☐ Asparagus
- ☐ Beet Greens
- ☐ Cabbage
- ☐ Celery
- ☐ Chard
- ☐ Cucumber
- ☐ Fennel
- ☐ Lettuce
- ☐ Onions
- ☐ Radishes
- ☐ Spinach
- ☐ Tomatoes
- ☐ Other: _____
- ☐ Other: _____
- ☐ Other: _____

Calories: _____

Fruit:
- ☐ Strawberries
- ☐ ½ Grapefruit
- ☐ Apple
- ☐ Orange
- ☐ Other: _____

Starch:
- ☐ Grissini
- ☐ Melba
- ☐ Other: _____

Calories: _____

Other:
- ☐ TBS. Milk
- ☐ Juice of 1 Lemon
- ☐ Stevia
- ☐ Shirataki/Miracle Noodles
- ☐ Other: _____
- ☐ Other: _____
- ☐ Other: _____

Calories: _____

VLCD **1** (Date): _____

WEIGHT: _____

HCG DOSAGE: _____

HUNGER LEVEL: _____

BEDTIME/WAKE TIME: _____

HOURS SLEEP: _____

TOTAL CALORIES: _____

SUPPLEMENTS: _____

☐ Multivitamin ☐ B12 Shot ☐ Lipo Shot

FELLOW HCGER TIP:

Sprinkling cinnamon & stevia on your P2 apple slices is the bomb.

INJECTION LOCATION TIME: _____

☐ Belly ☐ Deltoid ☐ Thigh ☐ Other: _____

DROPS / PELLETS DOSE TIMING

1st Dose: _____ 2nd Dose: _____

3rd Dose: _____ 4th Dose: _____

PERSONAL NOTES

· ·

....

....

....

....

....

....

....

LIQUIDS:

4 LITERS	128 oz = 1 GALLON
3.5 LITERS	120 oz
3 LITERS	112 oz
2.5 LITERS	104 oz
2 LITERS	96 oz = 3 QUARTS
1.5 LITERS	88 oz
1 LITER	80 oz
.5 LITERS	72 oz
	64 oz = 2 QUARTS
	56 oz
	48 oz
	40 oz
	32 oz = 1 QUART
	24 oz
	16 oz
	8 oz = 1 CUP

BREAKFAST   Time :

· ·

☐ None ☐ Fruit: _____ ☐ Protein: _____ Calories: _____

Serving Size: _____ Serving Size: _____

LUNCH Time :   WAS AN ITEM EATEN AS A SNACK? WHICH?   Time:

Protein:
- ☐ Chicken breast
- ☐ Beef
- ☐ Veal
- ☐ Shrimp
- ☐ Lobster
- ☐ White fish: _____
- ☐ Protein Shake
- ☐ Other: _____

Serving Size:
- ☐ 100 grams/3.5 oz
- ☐ Other: _____

Calories: _____

Vegetable:
- ☐ Asparagus
- ☐ Beet Greens
- ☐ Cabbage
- ☐ Celery
- ☐ Chard
- ☐ Cucumber
- ☐ Fennel
- ☐ Lettuce
- ☐ Onions
- ☐ Radishes
- ☐ Spinach
- ☐ Tomatoes
- ☐ Other: _____
- ☐ Other: _____
- ☐ Other: _____

Calories: _____

Fruit:
- ☐ Strawberries
- ☐ ½ Grapefruit
- ☐ Apple
- ☐ Orange
- ☐ Other: _____

Starch:
- ☐ Grissini
- ☐ Melba
- ☐ Other: _____

Calories: _____

Other:
- ☐ TBS. Milk
- ☐ Juice of 1 Lemon
- ☐ Stevia
- ☐ Shirataki/Miracle Noodles
- ☐ Other: _____
- ☐ Other: _____
- ☐ Other: _____

Calories: _____

DINNER Time :   WAS AN ITEM EATEN AS A SNACK? WHICH?   Time:

Protein:
- ☐ Chicken
- ☐ Beef
- ☐ Veal
- ☐ Shrimp
- ☐ Lobster
- ☐ White fish: _____
- ☐ Protein Shake
- ☐ Other: _____

Serving Size:
- ☐ 100 grams
- ☐ Other: _____

Calories: _____

Vegetable:
- ☐ Asparagus
- ☐ Beet Greens
- ☐ Cabbage
- ☐ Celery
- ☐ Chard
- ☐ Cucumber
- ☐ Fennel
- ☐ Lettuce
- ☐ Onions
- ☐ Radishes
- ☐ Spinach
- ☐ Tomatoes
- ☐ Other: _____
- ☐ Other: _____
- ☐ Other: _____

Calories: _____

Fruit:
- ☐ Strawberries
- ☐ ½ Grapefruit
- ☐ Apple
- ☐ Orange
- ☐ Other: _____

Starch:
- ☐ Grissini
- ☐ Melba
- ☐ Other: _____

Calories: _____

Other:
- ☐ TBS. Milk
- ☐ Juice of 1 Lemon
- ☐ Stevia
- ☐ Shirataki/Miracle Noodles
- ☐ Other: _____
- ☐ Other: _____
- ☐ Other: _____

Calories: _____

VLCD 2 (Date): _____

Success means doing the best we can with what we have. Success is THE DOING, not the getting; in THE TRYING, not the triumph. Success is a personal standard, reaching for the highest that is in us, becoming all that we can be.
— Zig Ziglar

WEIGHT: _____

HCG DOSAGE: _____

HUNGER LEVEL: _____

BEDTIME/WAKE TIME: _____

HOURS SLEEP: _____

TOTAL CALORIES: _____

SUPPLEMENTS: _____

☐ Multivitamin   ☐ B12 Shot   ☐ Lipo Shot

INJECTION LOCATION   TIME: _____

☐ Belly   ☐ Deltoid   ☐ Thigh   ☐ Other: _____

DROPS / PELLETS DOSE TIMING

1st Dose: _____   2nd Dose: _____
3rd Dose: _____   4th Dose: _____

PERSONAL NOTES

....
....
....
....
....
....

LIQUIDS:

4 LITERS	128 oz = 1 GALLON
3.5 LITERS	120 oz
3 LITERS	112 oz
2.5 LITERS	104 oz
2 LITERS	96 oz = 3 QUARTS
1.5 LITERS	88 oz
1 LITER	80 oz
.5 LITERS	72 oz
	64 oz = 2 QUARTS
	56 oz
	48 oz
	40 oz
	32 oz = 1 QUART
	24 oz
	16 oz
	8 oz = 1 CUP

BREAKFAST   Time :

☐ None   ☐ Fruit: _____   ☐ Protein: _____   Calories: _____
        Serving Size: _____   Serving Size: _____

LUNCH Time : 　　　　WAS AN ITEM EATEN AS A SNACK? WHICH?　　　　Time:

Protein:
- ☐ Chicken breast
- ☐ Beef
- ☐ Veal
- ☐ Shrimp
- ☐ Lobster
- ☐ White fish: _____
- ☐ Protein Shake
- ☐ Other: _____

Serving Size:
- ☐ 100 grams/3.5 oz
- ☐ Other: _____

Vegetable:
- ☐ Asparagus
- ☐ Beet Greens
- ☐ Cabbage
- ☐ Celery
- ☐ Chard
- ☐ Cucumber
- ☐ Fennel
- ☐ Lettuce
- ☐ Onions
- ☐ Radishes
- ☐ Spinach
- ☐ Tomatoes
- ☐ Other: _____
- ☐ Other: _____
- ☐ Other: _____

Fruit:
- ☐ Strawberries
- ☐ ½ Grapefruit
- ☐ Apple
- ☐ Orange
- ☐ Other: _____

Starch:
- ☐ Grissini
- ☐ Melba
- ☐ Other: _____

Other:
- ☐ TBS. Milk
- ☐ Juice of 1 Lemon
- ☐ Stevia
- ☐ Shirataki/Miracle Noodles
- ☐ Other: _____
- ☐ Other: _____
- ☐ Other: _____

Calories: _____   Calories: _____   Calories: _____   Calories: _____

DINNER Time : 　　　　WAS AN ITEM EATEN AS A SNACK? WHICH?　　　　Time:

Protein:
- ☐ Chicken
- ☐ Beef
- ☐ Veal
- ☐ Shrimp
- ☐ Lobster
- ☐ White fish: _____
- ☐ Protein Shake
- ☐ Other: _____

Serving Size:
- ☐ 100 grams
- ☐ Other: _____

Vegetable:
- ☐ Asparagus
- ☐ Beet Greens
- ☐ Cabbage
- ☐ Celery
- ☐ Chard
- ☐ Cucumber
- ☐ Fennel
- ☐ Lettuce
- ☐ Onions
- ☐ Radishes
- ☐ Spinach
- ☐ Tomatoes
- ☐ Other: _____
- ☐ Other: _____
- ☐ Other: _____

Fruit:
- ☐ Strawberries
- ☐ ½ Grapefruit
- ☐ Apple
- ☐ Orange
- ☐ Other: _____

Starch:
- ☐ Grissini
- ☐ Melba
- ☐ Other: _____

Other:
- ☐ TBS. Milk
- ☐ Juice of 1 Lemon
- ☐ Stevia
- ☐ Shirataki/Miracle Noodles
- ☐ Other: _____
- ☐ Other: _____
- ☐ Other: _____

Calories: _____   Calories: _____   Calories: _____   Calories: _____

VLCD 3 (Date): _____

FELLOW HCGER TIP:
Delicious Gingery Soup
Shave slices of fresh ginger, cherry tomatoes, and chicken or shrimp into homemade chicken de-fatted broth.

WEIGHT: _____

HCG DOSAGE: _____

HUNGER LEVEL: _____

BEDTIME/WAKE TIME: _____

HOURS SLEEP: _____

TOTAL CALORIES: _____

SUPPLEMENTS: _____

☐ Multivitamin   ☐ B12 Shot   ☐ Lipo Shot

INJECTION LOCATION   TIME: _____

☐ Belly   ☐ Deltoid   ☐ Thigh   ☐ Other: _____

DROPS / PELLETS DOSE TIMING

1st Dose: _____   2nd Dose: _____

3rd Dose: _____   4th Dose: _____

PERSONAL NOTES

....

....

....

....

....

....

....

LIQUIDS:

4 LITERS	128 oz = 1 GALLON
3.5 LITERS	120 oz
3 LITERS	112 oz
2.5 LITERS	104 oz
2 LITERS	96 oz = 3 QUARTS
1.5 LITERS	88 oz
1 LITER	80 oz
.5 LITERS	72 oz
	64 oz = 2 QUARTS
	56 oz
	48 oz
	40 oz
	32 oz = 1 QUART
	24 oz
	16 oz
	8 oz = 1 CUP

BREAKFAST   Time :

☐ None   ☐ Fruit: _____   ☐ Protein: _____   Calories: _____

Serving Size: _____   Serving Size: _____

LUNCH Time : 　　WAS AN ITEM EATEN AS A SNACK? WHICH?　　Time:

Protein:
- ☐ Chicken breast
- ☐ Beef
- ☐ Veal
- ☐ Shrimp
- ☐ Lobster
- ☐ White fish: _____
- ☐ Protein Shake
- ☐ Other: _____

Serving Size:
- ☐ 100 grams/3.5 oz
- ☐ Other: _____

Calories: _____

Vegetable:
- ☐ Asparagus
- ☐ Beet Greens
- ☐ Cabbage
- ☐ Celery
- ☐ Chard
- ☐ Cucumber
- ☐ Fennel
- ☐ Lettuce
- ☐ Onions
- ☐ Radishes
- ☐ Spinach
- ☐ Tomatoes
- ☐ Other: _____
- ☐ Other: _____
- ☐ Other: _____

Calories: _____

Fruit:
- ☐ Strawberries
- ☐ ½ Grapefruit
- ☐ Apple
- ☐ Orange
- ☐ Other: _____

Starch:
- ☐ Grissini
- ☐ Melba
- ☐ Other: _____

Calories: _____

Other:
- ☐ TBS. Milk
- ☐ Juice of 1 Lemon
- ☐ Stevia
- ☐ Shirataki/Miracle Noodles
- ☐ Other: _____
- ☐ Other: _____
- ☐ Other: _____

Calories: _____

DINNER Time : 　　WAS AN ITEM EATEN AS A SNACK? WHICH?　　Time:

Protein:
- ☐ Chicken
- ☐ Beef
- ☐ Veal
- ☐ Shrimp
- ☐ Lobster
- ☐ White fish: _____
- ☐ Protein Shake
- ☐ Other: _____

Serving Size:
- ☐ 100 grams
- ☐ Other: _____

Calories: _____

Vegetable:
- ☐ Asparagus
- ☐ Beet Greens
- ☐ Cabbage
- ☐ Celery
- ☐ Chard
- ☐ Cucumber
- ☐ Fennel
- ☐ Lettuce
- ☐ Onions
- ☐ Radishes
- ☐ Spinach
- ☐ Tomatoes
- ☐ Other: _____
- ☐ Other: _____
- ☐ Other: _____

Calories: _____

Fruit:
- ☐ Strawberries
- ☐ ½ Grapefruit
- ☐ Apple
- ☐ Orange
- ☐ Other: _____

Starch:
- ☐ Grissini
- ☐ Melba
- ☐ Other: _____

Calories: _____

Other:
- ☐ TBS. Milk
- ☐ Juice of 1 Lemon
- ☐ Stevia
- ☐ Shirataki/Miracle Noodles
- ☐ Other: _____
- ☐ Other: _____
- ☐ Other: _____

Calories: _____

VLCD 4 (Date): _____

Plan your hours to be productive, plan your weeks to be educational, plan your years to be purposeful, plan your life to be an experience of growth. *Plan to change.* PLAN TO GROW.
- Iyanla Vanzant

WEIGHT: _____

HCG DOSAGE: _____

HUNGER LEVEL: _____

BEDTIME/WAKE TIME: _____

HOURS SLEEP: _____

TOTAL CALORIES: _____

SUPPLEMENTS: _____

☐ Multivitamin   ☐ B12 Shot   ☐ Lipo Shot

INJECTION LOCATION   TIME: _____

☐ Belly   ☐ Deltoid   ☐ Thigh   ☐ Other: _____

DROPS / PELLETS DOSE TIMING

1st Dose: _____   2nd Dose: _____
3rd Dose: _____   4th Dose: _____

PERSONAL NOTES

....
....
....
....
....
....
....

LIQUIDS:

4 LITERS	128 oz = 1 GALLON
3.5 LITERS	120 oz
3 LITERS	112 oz
2.5 LITERS	104 oz
2 LITERS	96 oz = 3 QUARTS
1.5 LITERS	88 oz
1 LITER	80 oz
.5 LITERS	72 oz
	64 oz = 2 QUARTS
	56 oz
	48 oz
	40 oz
	32 oz = 1 QUART
	24 oz
	16 oz
	8 oz = 1 CUP

BREAKFAST   Time :

☐ None   ☐ Fruit: _____   ☐ Protein: _____   Calories: _____

Serving Size: _____   Serving Size: _____

LUNCH Time :   WAS AN ITEM EATEN AS A SNACK? WHICH?   Time:

Protein:
- ☐ Chicken breast
- ☐ Beef
- ☐ Veal
- ☐ Shrimp
- ☐ Lobster
- ☐ White fish: _____
- ☐ Protein Shake
- ☐ Other: _____

Serving Size:
- ☐ 100 grams/3.5 oz
- ☐ Other: _____

Vegetable:
- ☐ Asparagus
- ☐ Beet Greens
- ☐ Cabbage
- ☐ Celery
- ☐ Chard
- ☐ Cucumber
- ☐ Fennel
- ☐ Lettuce
- ☐ Onions
- ☐ Radishes
- ☐ Spinach
- ☐ Tomatoes
- ☐ Other: _____
- ☐ Other: _____
- ☐ Other: _____

Fruit:
- ☐ Strawberries
- ☐ ½ Grapefruit
- ☐ Apple
- ☐ Orange
- ☐ Other: _____

Starch:
- ☐ Grissini
- ☐ Melba
- ☐ Other: _____

Other:
- ☐ TBS. Milk
- ☐ Juice of 1 Lemon
- ☐ Stevia
- ☐ Shirataki/Miracle Noodles
- ☐ Other: _____
- ☐ Other: _____
- ☐ Other: _____

Calories: _____   Calories: _____   Calories: _____   Calories: _____

DINNER Time :   WAS AN ITEM EATEN AS A SNACK? WHICH?   Time:

Protein:
- ☐ Chicken
- ☐ Beef
- ☐ Veal
- ☐ Shrimp
- ☐ Lobster
- ☐ White fish: _____
- ☐ Protein Shake
- ☐ Other: _____

Serving Size:
- ☐ 100 grams
- ☐ Other: _____

Vegetable:
- ☐ Asparagus
- ☐ Beet Greens
- ☐ Cabbage
- ☐ Celery
- ☐ Chard
- ☐ Cucumber
- ☐ Fennel
- ☐ Lettuce
- ☐ Onions
- ☐ Radishes
- ☐ Spinach
- ☐ Tomatoes
- ☐ Other: _____
- ☐ Other: _____
- ☐ Other: _____

Fruit:
- ☐ Strawberries
- ☐ ½ Grapefruit
- ☐ Apple
- ☐ Orange
- ☐ Other: _____

Starch:
- ☐ Grissini
- ☐ Melba
- ☐ Other: _____

Other:
- ☐ TBS. Milk
- ☐ Juice of 1 Lemon
- ☐ Stevia
- ☐ Shirataki/Miracle Noodles
- ☐ Other: _____
- ☐ Other: _____
- ☐ Other: _____

Calories: _____   Calories: _____   Calories: _____   Calories: _____

VLCD **5** (Date): _____

WEIGHT: _____

HCG DOSAGE: _____

HUNGER LEVEL: _____

BEDTIME/WAKE TIME: _____

HOURS SLEEP: _____

TOTAL CALORIES: _____

SUPPLEMENTS: _____

☐ Multivitamin ☐ B12 Shot ☐ Lipo Shot

FELLOW HCGER TIP:

Flavored teas...

with stevia, can save you. No joke. When choosing one, just double check ingredients as some acually contain juice - not a good idea.

INJECTION LOCATION   TIME: _____

☐ Belly ☐ Deltoid ☐ Thigh ☐ Other: _____

DROPS / PELLETS DOSE TIMING

1st Dose: _____   2nd Dose: _____

3rd Dose: _____   4th Dose: _____

PERSONAL NOTES

....

....

....

....

....

....

....

LIQUIDS:

4 LITERS	128 oz = 1 GALLON
3.5 LITERS	120 oz
3 LITERS	112 oz
2.5 LITERS	104 oz
2 LITERS	96 oz = 3 QUARTS
1.5 LITERS	88 oz
1 LITER	80 oz
.5 LITERS	72 oz
	64 oz = 2 QUARTS
	56 oz
	48 oz
	40 oz
	32 oz = 1 QUART
	24 oz
	16 oz
	8 oz = 1 CUP

BREAKFAST   Time :

☐ None ☐ Fruit: _____   ☐ Protein: _____   Calories: _____

Serving Size: _____   Serving Size: _____

LUNCH Time :   WAS AN ITEM EATEN AS A SNACK? WHICH?   Time:

Protein:
- [ ] Chicken breast
- [ ] Beef
- [ ] Veal
- [ ] Shrimp
- [ ] Lobster
- [ ] White fish: _____
- [ ] Protein Shake
- [ ] Other: _____

Serving Size:
- [ ] 100 grams/3.5 oz
- [ ] Other: _____

Vegetable:
- [ ] Asparagus
- [ ] Beet Greens
- [ ] Cabbage
- [ ] Celery
- [ ] Chard
- [ ] Cucumber
- [ ] Fennel
- [ ] Lettuce
- [ ] Onions
- [ ] Radishes
- [ ] Spinach
- [ ] Tomatoes
- [ ] Other: _____
- [ ] Other: _____
- [ ] Other: _____

Fruit:
- [ ] Strawberries
- [ ] ½ Grapefruit
- [ ] Apple
- [ ] Orange
- [ ] Other: _____

Starch:
- [ ] Grissini
- [ ] Melba
- [ ] Other: _____

Other:
- [ ] TBS. Milk
- [ ] Juice of 1 Lemon
- [ ] Stevia
- [ ] Shirataki/Miracle Noodles
- [ ] Other: _____
- [ ] Other: _____
- [ ] Other: _____

Calories: _____   Calories: _____   Calories: _____   Calories: _____

DINNER Time :   WAS AN ITEM EATEN AS A SNACK? WHICH?   Time:

Protein:
- [ ] Chicken
- [ ] Beef
- [ ] Veal
- [ ] Shrimp
- [ ] Lobster
- [ ] White fish: _____
- [ ] Protein Shake
- [ ] Other: _____

Serving Size:
- [ ] 100 grams
- [ ] Other: _____

Vegetable:
- [ ] Asparagus
- [ ] Beet Greens
- [ ] Cabbage
- [ ] Celery
- [ ] Chard
- [ ] Cucumber
- [ ] Fennel
- [ ] Lettuce
- [ ] Onions
- [ ] Radishes
- [ ] Spinach
- [ ] Tomatoes
- [ ] Other: _____
- [ ] Other: _____
- [ ] Other: _____

Fruit:
- [ ] Strawberries
- [ ] ½ Grapefruit
- [ ] Apple
- [ ] Orange
- [ ] Other: _____

Starch:
- [ ] Grissini
- [ ] Melba
- [ ] Other: _____

Other:
- [ ] TBS. Milk
- [ ] Juice of 1 Lemon
- [ ] Stevia
- [ ] Shirataki/Miracle Noodles
- [ ] Other: _____
- [ ] Other: _____
- [ ] Other: _____

Calories: _____   Calories: _____   Calories: _____   Calories: _____

VLCD **6** (Date): _____

WEIGHT: _____

HCG DOSAGE: _____

HUNGER LEVEL: _____

BEDTIME/WAKE TIME: _____

HOURS SLEEP: _____

TOTAL CALORIES: _____

SUPPLEMENTS: _____

☐ Multivitamin   ☐ B12 Shot   ☐ Lipo Shot

> When you're trying to motivate yourself, *appreciate* the fact that you're even **THINKING** about making a change. And as you move forward, **ALLOW** yourself to be good enough.
> — Alice Domar

INJECTION LOCATION   TIME: _____

☐ Belly   ☐ Deltoid   ☐ Thigh   ☐ Other: _____

DROPS / PELLETS DOSE TIMING

1st Dose: _____   2nd Dose: _____

3rd Dose: _____   4th Dose: _____

PERSONAL NOTES

....

....

....

....

....

....

....

LIQUIDS:

4 LITERS	128 oz = 1 GALLON
3.5 LITERS	120 oz
3 LITERS	112 oz
2.5 LITERS	104 oz
2 LITERS	96 oz = 3 QUART
1.5 LITERS	88 oz
1 LITER	80 oz
.5 LITERS	72 oz
	64 oz = 2 QUARTS
	56 oz
	48 oz
	40 oz
	32 oz = 1 QUART
	24 oz
	16 oz
	8 oz = 1 CUP

BREAKFAST   Time: _____

☐ None   ☐ Fruit: _____   ☐ Protein: _____   Calories: _____

Serving Size: _____   Serving Size: _____

LUNCH Time :

Protein:
- [ ] Chicken breast
- [ ] Beef
- [ ] Veal
- [ ] Shrimp
- [ ] Lobster
- [ ] White fish: _____
- [ ] Protein Shake
- [ ] Other: _____

Serving Size:
- [ ] 100 grams/3.5 oz
- [ ] Other: _____

Calories: _____

Vegetable:
- [ ] Asparagus
- [ ] Beet Greens
- [ ] Cabbage
- [ ] Celery
- [ ] Chard
- [ ] Cucumber
- [ ] Fennel
- [ ] Lettuce
- [ ] Onions
- [ ] Radishes
- [ ] Spinach
- [ ] Tomatoes
- [ ] Other: _____
- [ ] Other: _____
- [ ] Other: _____

Calories: _____

Fruit:
- [ ] Strawberries
- [ ] ½ Grapefruit
- [ ] Apple
- [ ] Orange
- [ ] Other: _____

Starch:
- [ ] Grissini
- [ ] Melba
- [ ] Other: _____

Calories: _____

Other:
- [ ] TBS. Milk
- [ ] Juice of 1 Lemon
- [ ] Stevia
- [ ] Shirataki/Miracle Noodles
- [ ] Other: _____
- [ ] Other: _____
- [ ] Other: _____

Calories: _____

DINNER Time :

Protein:
- [ ] Chicken
- [ ] Beef
- [ ] Veal
- [ ] Shrimp
- [ ] Lobster
- [ ] White fish: _____
- [ ] Protein Shake
- [ ] Other: _____

Serving Size:
- [ ] 100 grams
- [ ] Other: _____

Calories: _____

Vegetable:
- [ ] Asparagus
- [ ] Beet Greens
- [ ] Cabbage
- [ ] Celery
- [ ] Chard
- [ ] Cucumber
- [ ] Fennel
- [ ] Lettuce
- [ ] Onions
- [ ] Radishes
- [ ] Spinach
- [ ] Tomatoes
- [ ] Other: _____
- [ ] Other: _____
- [ ] Other: _____

Calories: _____

Fruit:
- [ ] Strawberries
- [ ] ½ Grapefruit
- [ ] Apple
- [ ] Orange
- [ ] Other: _____

Starch:
- [ ] Grissini
- [ ] Melba
- [ ] Other: _____

Calories: _____

Other:
- [ ] TBS. Milk
- [ ] Juice of 1 Lemon
- [ ] Stevia
- [ ] Shirataki/Miracle Noodles
- [ ] Other: _____
- [ ] Other: _____
- [ ] Other: _____

Calories: _____

VLCD 7 (Date): _____

FELLOW HCGER TIP:

Go-to Breakfast Smoothie

Strawberries, whizzed with ice, water, stevia and 1 tbs. milk. Put in a takeout bottle to go.

WEIGHT: _____

HCG DOSAGE: _____

HUNGER LEVEL: _____

BEDTIME/WAKE TIME: _____

HOURS SLEEP: _____

TOTAL CALORIES: _____

SUPPLEMENTS: _____

☐ Multivitamin   ☐ B12 Shot   ☐ Lipo Shot

INJECTION LOCATION   TIME: _____

☐ Belly   ☐ Deltoid   ☐ Thigh   ☐ Other: _____

DROPS / PELLETS DOSE TIMING

1st Dose: _____   2nd Dose: _____

3rd Dose: _____   4th Dose: _____

LIQUIDS:

4 LITERS	128 oz = 1 GALLON
3.5 LITERS	120 oz
3 LITERS	112 oz
2.5 LITERS	104 oz
2 LITERS	96 oz = 3 QUARTS
1.5 LITERS	88 oz
1 LITER	80 oz
.5 LITERS	72 oz
	64 oz = 2 QUARTS
	56 oz
	48 oz
	40 oz
	32 oz = 1 QUART
	24 oz
	16 oz
	8 oz = 1 CUP

PERSONAL NOTES

....

....

....

....

....

....

....

BREAKFAST   Time: _____

☐ None   ☐ Fruit: _____   ☐ Protein: _____   Calories: _____

Serving Size: _____   Serving Size: _____

LUNCH Time :   WAS AN ITEM EATEN AS A SNACK? WHICH?   Time:

Protein:
- ☐ Chicken breast
- ☐ Beef
- ☐ Veal
- ☐ Shrimp
- ☐ Lobster
- ☐ White fish: _____
- ☐ Protein Shake
- ☐ Other: _____

Serving Size:
- ☐ 100 grams/3.5 oz
- ☐ Other: _____

Vegetable:
- ☐ Asparagus
- ☐ Beet Greens
- ☐ Cabbage
- ☐ Celery
- ☐ Chard
- ☐ Cucumber
- ☐ Fennel
- ☐ Lettuce
- ☐ Onions
- ☐ Radishes
- ☐ Spinach
- ☐ Tomatoes
- ☐ Other: _____
- ☐ Other: _____
- ☐ Other: _____

Fruit:
- ☐ Strawberries
- ☐ ½ Grapefruit
- ☐ Apple
- ☐ Orange
- ☐ Other: _____

Starch:
- ☐ Grissini
- ☐ Melba
- ☐ Other: _____

Other:
- ☐ TBS. Milk
- ☐ Juice of 1 Lemon
- ☐ Stevia
- ☐ Shirataki/Miracle Noodles
- ☐ Other: _____
- ☐ Other: _____
- ☐ Other: _____

Calories: _____   Calories: _____   Calories: _____   Calories: _____

DINNER Time :   WAS AN ITEM EATEN AS A SNACK? WHICH?   Time:

Protein:
- ☐ Chicken
- ☐ Beef
- ☐ Veal
- ☐ Shrimp
- ☐ Lobster
- ☐ White fish: _____
- ☐ Protein Shake
- ☐ Other: _____

Serving Size:
- ☐ 100 grams
- ☐ Other: _____

Vegetable:
- ☐ Asparagus
- ☐ Beet Greens
- ☐ Cabbage
- ☐ Celery
- ☐ Chard
- ☐ Cucumber
- ☐ Fennel
- ☐ Lettuce
- ☐ Onions
- ☐ Radishes
- ☐ Spinach
- ☐ Tomatoes
- ☐ Other: _____
- ☐ Other: _____
- ☐ Other: _____

Fruit:
- ☐ Strawberries
- ☐ ½ Grapefruit
- ☐ Apple
- ☐ Orange
- ☐ Other: _____

Starch:
- ☐ Grissini
- ☐ Melba
- ☐ Other: _____

Other:
- ☐ TBS. Milk
- ☐ Juice of 1 Lemon
- ☐ Stevia
- ☐ Shirataki/Miracle Noodles
- ☐ Other: _____
- ☐ Other: _____
- ☐ Other: _____

Calories: _____   Calories: _____   Calories: _____   Calories: _____

Reflections ON WEEK 1

REMEMBER, THIS IS NOT JUST ABOUT LOSING WEIGHT. IT'S ABOUT CHANGING YOUR WHOLE MINDSET ABOUT FOOD AND YOUR BODY,

YOU ARE BREAKING OLD PATTERNS RIGHT NOW. YOU ARE CREATING NEW PATTERNS. TRY NOT TO FOCUS YOUR PROGESS SOLELY ON WEIGHT LOSS.

SO WITH THAT IN MIND, HOW DID THIS WEEK GO?

What are you proud of? Why are you proud of it? What did you struggle with? What would you like to work on changing? What specific logical ways can you think of to make those adjustments? Or maybe you're just burned out at the moment - it's okay to just make it a rant.

....
....
....
....
....
....
....
....
....
....
....
....
....
....
....
....
....

Week 2

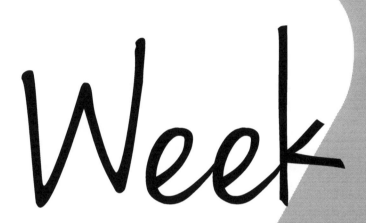

"IN MY EXPERIENCE, nothing worthwhile has ever been all that easy. But it certainly has been worthwhile, regardless how difficult it seemed."

– Robert Fanney

VLCD **8** (Date): _____

WEIGHT: _____

HCG DOSAGE: _____

HUNGER LEVEL: _____

BEDTIME/WAKE TIME: _____

HOURS SLEEP: _____

TOTAL CALORIES: _____

SUPPLEMENTS: _____

☐ Multivitamin ☐ B12 Shot ☐ Lipo Shot

> When I remove the layers that say I can't, I *discover* A BURNING EMBER that says I SHOULD, I CAN, AND I WILL.
> — *Charles F. Glassman*

INJECTION LOCATION   TIME: _____

☐ Belly ☐ Deltoid ☐ Thigh ☐ Other: _____

DROPS / PELLETS DOSE TIMING

1st Dose: _____   2nd Dose: _____

3rd Dose: _____   4th Dose: _____

PERSONAL NOTES

....

....

....

....

....

....

....

LIQUIDS:

4 LITERS		128 oz = 1 GALLON
3.5 LITERS		120 oz
3 LITERS		112 oz
2.5 LITERS		104 oz
2 LITERS		96 oz = 3 QUARTS
1.5 LITERS		88 oz
1 LITER		80 oz
.5 LITERS		72 oz
		64 oz = 2 QUARTS
		56 oz
		48 oz
		40 oz
		32 oz = 1 QUART
		24 oz
		16 oz
		8 oz = 1 CUP

BREAKFAST   Time :

☐ None ☐ Fruit: _____ ☐ Protein: _____   Calories: _____

Serving Size: _____   Serving Size: _____

LUNCH Time :
Time:

Protein:
- ☐ Chicken breast
- ☐ Beef
- ☐ Veal
- ☐ Shrimp
- ☐ Lobster
- ☐ White fish: _____
- ☐ Protein Shake
- ☐ Other: _____

Serving Size:
- ☐ 100 grams/3.5 oz
- ☐ Other: _____

Calories: _____

Vegetable:
- ☐ Asparagus
- ☐ Beet Greens
- ☐ Cabbage
- ☐ Celery
- ☐ Chard
- ☐ Cucumber
- ☐ Fennel
- ☐ Lettuce
- ☐ Onions
- ☐ Radishes
- ☐ Spinach
- ☐ Tomatoes
- ☐ Other: _____
- ☐ Other: _____
- ☐ Other: _____

Calories: _____

Fruit:
- ☐ Strawberries
- ☐ ½ Grapefruit
- ☐ Apple
- ☐ Orange
- ☐ Other: _____

Starch:
- ☐ Grissini
- ☐ Melba
- ☐ Other: _____

Calories: _____

Other:
- ☐ TBS. Milk
- ☐ Juice of 1 Lemon
- ☐ Stevia
- ☐ Shirataki/Miracle Noodles
- ☐ Other: _____
- ☐ Other: _____
- ☐ Other: _____

Calories: _____

DINNER Time :
Time:

Protein:
- ☐ Chicken
- ☐ Beef
- ☐ Veal
- ☐ Shrimp
- ☐ Lobster
- ☐ White fish: _____
- ☐ Protein Shake
- ☐ Other: _____

Serving Size:
- ☐ 100 grams
- ☐ Other: _____

Calories: _____

Vegetable:
- ☐ Asparagus
- ☐ Beet Greens
- ☐ Cabbage
- ☐ Celery
- ☐ Chard
- ☐ Cucumber
- ☐ Fennel
- ☐ Lettuce
- ☐ Onions
- ☐ Radishes
- ☐ Spinach
- ☐ Tomatoes
- ☐ Other: _____
- ☐ Other: _____
- ☐ Other: _____

Calories: _____

Fruit:
- ☐ Strawberries
- ☐ ½ Grapefruit
- ☐ Apple
- ☐ Orange
- ☐ Other: _____

Starch:
- ☐ Grissini
- ☐ Melba
- ☐ Other: _____

Calories: _____

Other:
- ☐ TBS. Milk
- ☐ Juice of 1 Lemon
- ☐ Stevia
- ☐ Shirataki/Miracle Noodles
- ☐ Other: _____
- ☐ Other: _____
- ☐ Other: _____

Calories: _____

FELLOW HCGER TIP:

Social Settings

"If I'm ever going to be around other people eating during Phase 2, I make *sure* to BRING SOMETHING TO EAT *and* SOMETHING TO DRINK."

WEIGHT: _____

HCG DOSAGE: _____

HUNGER LEVEL: _____

BEDTIME/WAKE TIME: _____

HOURS SLEEP: _____

TOTAL CALORIES: _____

SUPPLEMENTS: _____

☐ Multivitamin   ☐ B12 Shot   ☐ Lipo Shot

INJECTION LOCATION   TIME: _____

☐ Belly   ☐ Deltoid   ☐ Thigh   ☐ Other: _____

DROPS / PELLETS DOSE TIMING

1st Dose: _____   2nd Dose: _____
3rd Dose: _____   4th Dose: _____

PERSONAL NOTES

....

....

....

....

....

....

....

LIQUIDS:

4 LITERS	128 oz = 1 GALLON
3.5 LITERS	120 oz
3 LITERS	112 oz
2.5 LITERS	104 oz
2 LITERS	96 oz = 3 QUARTS
1.5 LITERS	88 oz
1 LITER	80 oz
.5 LITERS	72 oz
	64 oz = 2 QUARTS
	56 oz
	48 oz
	40 oz
	32 oz = 1 QUART
	24 oz
	16 oz
	8 oz = 1 CUP

BREAKFAST   *Time :*

....

☐ None   ☐ Fruit: _____   ☐ Protein: _____   *Calories:* _____

Serving Size: _____   *Serving Size:* _____

LUNCH Time : _____

Protein:
- ☐ Chicken breast
- ☐ Beef
- ☐ Veal
- ☐ Shrimp
- ☐ Lobster
- ☐ White fish: _____
- ☐ Protein Shake
- ☐ Other: _____

Serving Size:
- ☐ 100 grams/3.5 oz
- ☐ Other: _____

Calories: _____

Vegetable:
- ☐ Asparagus
- ☐ Beet Greens
- ☐ Cabbage
- ☐ Celery
- ☐ Chard
- ☐ Cucumber
- ☐ Fennel
- ☐ Lettuce
- ☐ Onions
- ☐ Radishes
- ☐ Spinach
- ☐ Tomatoes
- ☐ Other: _____
- ☐ Other: _____
- ☐ Other: _____

Calories: _____

Fruit:
- ☐ Strawberries
- ☐ ½ Grapefruit
- ☐ Apple
- ☐ Orange
- ☐ Other: _____

Starch:
- ☐ Grissini
- ☐ Melba
- ☐ Other: _____

Calories: _____

Other:
- ☐ TBS. Milk
- ☐ Juice of 1 Lemon
- ☐ Stevia
- ☐ Shirataki/Miracle Noodles
- ☐ Other: _____
- ☐ Other: _____
- ☐ Other: _____

Calories: _____

DINNER Time : _____

Protein:
- ☐ Chicken
- ☐ Beef
- ☐ Veal
- ☐ Shrimp
- ☐ Lobster
- ☐ White fish: _____
- ☐ Protein Shake
- ☐ Other: _____

Serving Size:
- ☐ 100 grams
- ☐ Other: _____

Calories: _____

Vegetable:
- ☐ Asparagus
- ☐ Beet Greens
- ☐ Cabbage
- ☐ Celery
- ☐ Chard
- ☐ Cucumber
- ☐ Fennel
- ☐ Lettuce
- ☐ Onions
- ☐ Radishes
- ☐ Spinach
- ☐ Tomatoes
- ☐ Other: _____
- ☐ Other: _____
- ☐ Other: _____

Calories: _____

Fruit:
- ☐ Strawberries
- ☐ ½ Grapefruit
- ☐ Apple
- ☐ Orange
- ☐ Other: _____

Starch:
- ☐ Grissini
- ☐ Melba
- ☐ Other: _____

Calories: _____

Other:
- ☐ TBS. Milk
- ☐ Juice of 1 Lemon
- ☐ Stevia
- ☐ Shirataki/Miracle Noodles
- ☐ Other: _____
- ☐ Other: _____
- ☐ Other: _____

Calories: _____

VLCD 10 (Date): _____

WEIGHT: _____

HCG DOSAGE: _____

HUNGER LEVEL: _____

BEDTIME/WAKE TIME: _____

HOURS SLEEP: _____

TOTAL CALORIES: _____

SUPPLEMENTS: _____

☐ Multivitamin   ☐ B12 Shot   ☐ Lipo Shot

Don't let what you cannot do interfere WITH WHAT YOU CAN DO

- John Wooden

INJECTION LOCATION   TIME: _____

☐ Belly   ☐ Deltoid   ☐ Thigh   ☐ Other: _____

DROPS / PELLETS DOSE TIMING

1st Dose: _____   2nd Dose: _____

3rd Dose: _____   4th Dose: _____

PERSONAL NOTES

....

....

....

....

....

....

....

LIQUIDS:

4 LITERS	128 oz = 1 GALLON
3.5 LITERS	120 oz
3 LITERS	112 oz
2.5 LITERS	104 oz
2 LITERS	96 oz = 3 QUARTS
1.5 LITERS	88 oz
1 LITER	80 oz
.5 LITERS	72 oz
	64 oz = 2 QUARTS
	56 oz
	48 oz
	40 oz
	32 oz = 1 QUART
	24 oz
	16 oz
	8 oz = 1 CUP

BREAKFAST   Time :

☐ None   ☐ Fruit: _____   ☐ Protein: _____   Calories: _____

Serving Size: _____   Serving Size: _____

LUNCH Time :   WAS AN ITEM EATEN AS A SNACK? WHICH?   Time:

Protein:
- ☐ Chicken breast
- ☐ Beef
- ☐ Veal
- ☐ Shrimp
- ☐ Lobster
- ☐ White fish: _____
- ☐ Protein Shake
- ☐ Other: _____

Serving Size:
- ☐ 100 grams/3.5 oz
- ☐ Other: _____

Vegetable:
- ☐ Asparagus
- ☐ Beet Greens
- ☐ Cabbage
- ☐ Celery
- ☐ Chard
- ☐ Cucumber
- ☐ Fennel
- ☐ Lettuce
- ☐ Onions
- ☐ Radishes
- ☐ Spinach
- ☐ Tomatoes
- ☐ Other: _____
- ☐ Other: _____
- ☐ Other: _____

Fruit:
- ☐ Strawberries
- ☐ ½ Grapefruit
- ☐ Apple
- ☐ Orange
- ☐ Other: _____

Starch:
- ☐ Grissini
- ☐ Melba
- ☐ Other: _____

Other:
- ☐ TBS. Milk
- ☐ Juice of 1 Lemon
- ☐ Stevia
- ☐ Shirataki/Miracle Noodles
- ☐ Other: _____
- ☐ Other: _____
- ☐ Other: _____

Calories: _____   Calories: _____   Calories: _____   Calories: _____

DINNER Time :   WAS AN ITEM EATEN AS A SNACK? WHICH?   Time:

Protein:
- ☐ Chicken
- ☐ Beef
- ☐ Veal
- ☐ Shrimp
- ☐ Lobster
- ☐ White fish: _____
- ☐ Protein Shake
- ☐ Other: _____

Serving Size:
- ☐ 100 grams
- ☐ Other: _____

Vegetable:
- ☐ Asparagus
- ☐ Beet Greens
- ☐ Cabbage
- ☐ Celery
- ☐ Chard
- ☐ Cucumber
- ☐ Fennel
- ☐ Lettuce
- ☐ Onions
- ☐ Radishes
- ☐ Spinach
- ☐ Tomatoes
- ☐ Other: _____
- ☐ Other: _____
- ☐ Other: _____

Fruit:
- ☐ Strawberries
- ☐ ½ Grapefruit
- ☐ Apple
- ☐ Orange
- ☐ Other: _____

Starch:
- ☐ Grissini
- ☐ Melba
- ☐ Other: _____

Other:
- ☐ TBS. Milk
- ☐ Juice of 1 Lemon
- ☐ Stevia
- ☐ Shirataki/Miracle Noodles
- ☐ Other: _____
- ☐ Other: _____
- ☐ Other: _____

Calories: _____   Calories: _____   Calories: _____   Calories: _____

Accept Detox

Food addiction is real in my opinion. Understanding that your body may go through detox helps. This passes. On a hard day remember very soon it will feel easier.

VLCD 11 (Date): _____

WEIGHT: _____

HCG DOSAGE: _____

HUNGER LEVEL: _____

BEDTIME/WAKE TIME: _____

HOURS SLEEP: _____

TOTAL CALORIES: _____

SUPPLEMENTS: _____

☐ Multivitamin ☐ B12 Shot ☐ Lipo Shot

INJECTION LOCATION TIME: _____

☐ Belly ☐ Deltoid ☐ Thigh ☐ Other: _____

DROPS / PELLETS DOSE TIMING

1st Dose: _____ 2nd Dose: _____

3rd Dose: _____ 4th Dose: _____

PERSONAL NOTES

....

....

....

....

....

....

LIQUIDS:

4 LITERS	128 oz = 1 GALLON
3.5 LITERS	120 oz
3 LITERS	112 oz
2.5 LITERS	104 oz
2 LITERS	96 oz = 3 QUARTS
1.5 LITERS	88 oz
1 LITER	80 oz
.5 LITERS	72 oz
	64 oz = 2 QUARTS
	56 oz
	48 oz
	40 oz
	32 oz = 1 QUART
	24 oz
	16 oz
	8 oz = 1 CUP

BREAKFAST Time :

....

☐ None ☐ Fruit: _____ ☐ Protein: _____ Calories: _____

Serving Size: _____ Serving Size: _____

LUNCH Time : ___   WAS AN ITEM EATEN AS A SNACK? WHICH?   Time: ___

Protein:
- ☐ Chicken breast
- ☐ Beef
- ☐ Veal
- ☐ Shrimp
- ☐ Lobster
- ☐ White fish: _____
- ☐ Protein Shake
- ☐ Other: _____

Serving Size:
- ☐ 100 grams/3.5 oz
- ☐ Other: _____

Vegetable:
- ☐ Asparagus
- ☐ Beet Greens
- ☐ Cabbage
- ☐ Celery
- ☐ Chard
- ☐ Cucumber
- ☐ Fennel
- ☐ Lettuce
- ☐ Onions
- ☐ Radishes
- ☐ Spinach
- ☐ Tomatoes
- ☐ Other: _____
- ☐ Other: _____
- ☐ Other: _____

Fruit:
- ☐ Strawberries
- ☐ ½ Grapefruit
- ☐ Apple
- ☐ Orange
- ☐ Other: _____

Starch:
- ☐ Grissini
- ☐ Melba
- ☐ Other: _____

Other:
- ☐ TBS. Milk
- ☐ Juice of 1 Lemon
- ☐ Stevia
- ☐ Shirataki/Miracle Noodles
- ☐ Other: _____
- ☐ Other: _____
- ☐ Other: _____

Calories: _____   Calories: _____   Calories: _____   Calories: _____

DINNER Time : ___   WAS AN ITEM EATEN AS A SNACK? WHICH?   Time: ___

Protein:
- ☐ Chicken
- ☐ Beef
- ☐ Veal
- ☐ Shrimp
- ☐ Lobster
- ☐ White fish: _____
- ☐ Protein Shake
- ☐ Other: _____

Serving Size:
- ☐ 100 grams
- ☐ Other: _____

Vegetable:
- ☐ Asparagus
- ☐ Beet Greens
- ☐ Cabbage
- ☐ Celery
- ☐ Chard
- ☐ Cucumber
- ☐ Fennel
- ☐ Lettuce
- ☐ Onions
- ☐ Radishes
- ☐ Spinach
- ☐ Tomatoes
- ☐ Other: _____
- ☐ Other: _____
- ☐ Other: _____

Fruit:
- ☐ Strawberries
- ☐ ½ Grapefruit
- ☐ Apple
- ☐ Orange
- ☐ Other: _____

Starch:
- ☐ Grissini
- ☐ Melba
- ☐ Other: _____

Other:
- ☐ TBS. Milk
- ☐ Juice of 1 Lemon
- ☐ Stevia
- ☐ Shirataki/Miracle Noodles
- ☐ Other: _____
- ☐ Other: _____
- ☐ Other: _____

Calories: _____   Calories: _____   Calories: _____   Calories: _____

FELLOW HCGER TIP:

THE MAGIC OF *Bib Lettuce*

Butter/bib lettuce is great for making lettuce wraps filled with a P2 protein and thinly sliced P2 veggies.

VLCD 12 (Date): _____

WEIGHT: _____

HCG DOSAGE: _____

HUNGER LEVEL: _____

BEDTIME/WAKE TIME: _____

HOURS SLEEP: _____

TOTAL CALORIES: _____

SUPPLEMENTS: _____

☐ Multivitamin   ☐ B12 Shot   ☐ Lipo Shot

INJECTION LOCATION   TIME: _____

☐ Belly   ☐ Deltoid   ☐ Thigh   ☐ Other: _____

DROPS / PELLETS DOSE TIMING

1st Dose: _____   2nd Dose: _____

3rd Dose: _____   4th Dose: _____

PERSONAL NOTES

....

....

....

....

....

....

....

LIQUIDS:

4 LITERS	128 oz = 1 GALLON
3.5 LITERS	120 oz
3 LITERS	112 oz
2.5 LITERS	104 oz
2 LITERS	96 oz = 3 QUARTS
1.5 LITERS	88 oz
1 LITER	80 oz
.5 LITERS	72 oz
	64 oz = 2 QUARTS
	56 oz
	48 oz
	40 oz
	32 oz = 1 QUART
	24 oz
	16 oz
	8 oz = 1 CUP

BREAKFAST   Time :

☐ None   ☐ Fruit: _____   ☐ Protein: _____   Calories: _____

Serving Size: _____   Serving Size: _____

LUNCH Time :   WAS AN ITEM EATEN AS A SNACK? WHICH?   Time:

Protein:
- ☐ Chicken breast
- ☐ Beef
- ☐ Veal
- ☐ Shrimp
- ☐ Lobster
- ☐ White fish: _____
- ☐ Protein Shake
- ☐ Other: _____

Serving Size:
- ☐ 100 grams/3.5 oz
- ☐ Other: _____

Calories: _____

Vegetable:
- ☐ Asparagus
- ☐ Beet Greens
- ☐ Cabbage
- ☐ Celery
- ☐ Chard
- ☐ Cucumber
- ☐ Fennel
- ☐ Lettuce
- ☐ Onions
- ☐ Radishes
- ☐ Spinach
- ☐ Tomatoes
- ☐ Other: _____
- ☐ Other: _____
- ☐ Other: _____

Calories: _____

Fruit:
- ☐ Strawberries
- ☐ ½ Grapefruit
- ☐ Apple
- ☐ Orange
- ☐ Other: _____

Starch:
- ☐ Grissini
- ☐ Melba
- ☐ Other: _____

Calories: _____

Other:
- ☐ TBS. Milk
- ☐ Juice of 1 Lemon
- ☐ Stevia
- ☐ Shirataki/Miracle Noodles
- ☐ Other: _____
- ☐ Other: _____
- ☐ Other: _____

Calories: _____

DINNER Time :   WAS AN ITEM EATEN AS A SNACK? WHICH?   Time:

Protein:
- ☐ Chicken
- ☐ Beef
- ☐ Veal
- ☐ Shrimp
- ☐ Lobster
- ☐ White fish: _____
- ☐ Protein Shake
- ☐ Other: _____

Serving Size:
- ☐ 100 grams
- ☐ Other: _____

Calories: _____

Vegetable:
- ☐ Asparagus
- ☐ Beet Greens
- ☐ Cabbage
- ☐ Celery
- ☐ Chard
- ☐ Cucumber
- ☐ Fennel
- ☐ Lettuce
- ☐ Onions
- ☐ Radishes
- ☐ Spinach
- ☐ Tomatoes
- ☐ Other: _____
- ☐ Other: _____
- ☐ Other: _____

Calories: _____

Fruit:
- ☐ Strawberries
- ☐ ½ Grapefruit
- ☐ Apple
- ☐ Orange
- ☐ Other: _____

Starch:
- ☐ Grissini
- ☐ Melba
- ☐ Other: _____

Calories: _____

Other:
- ☐ TBS. Milk
- ☐ Juice of 1 Lemon
- ☐ Stevia
- ☐ Shirataki/Miracle Noodles
- ☐ Other: _____
- ☐ Other: _____
- ☐ Other: _____

Calories: _____

VLCD 13 (Date): _____

WEIGHT: _____

HCG DOSAGE: _____

HUNGER LEVEL: _____

BEDTIME/WAKE TIME: _____

HOURS SLEEP: _____

TOTAL CALORIES: _____

SUPPLEMENTS: _____

☐ Multivitamin   ☐ B12 Shot   ☐ Lipo Shot

When OBSTACLES ARISE, you change your direction to reach your *goal*; you DO NOT CHANGE YOUR DECISION to get there.
— Zig Ziglar

INJECTION LOCATION   TIME: _____

☐ Belly   ☐ Deltoid   ☐ Thigh   ☐ Other: _____

DROPS / PELLETS DOSE TIMING

1st Dose: _____   2nd Dose: _____

3rd Dose: _____   4th Dose: _____

PERSONAL NOTES

....

....

....

....

....

....

....

....

LIQUIDS:

4 LITERS	128 oz = 1 GALLON
3.5 LITERS	120 oz
3 LITERS	112 oz
2.5 LITERS	104 oz
2 LITERS	96 oz = 3 QUARTS
1.5 LITERS	88 oz
1 LITER	80 oz
.5 LITERS	72 oz
	64 oz = 2 QUARTS
	56 oz
	48 oz
	40 oz
	32 oz = 1 QUART
	24 oz
	16 oz
	8 oz = 1 CUP

BREAKFAST   Time :

☐ None   ☐ Fruit: _____   ☐ Protein: _____   *Calories:* _____

Serving Size: _____   Serving Size: _____

LUNCH Time : WAS AN ITEM EATEN AS A SNACK? WHICH? Time:

Protein:
- [ ] Chicken breast
- [ ] Beef
- [ ] Veal
- [ ] Shrimp
- [ ] Lobster
- [ ] White fish: _____
- [ ] Protein Shake
- [ ] Other: _____

Serving Size:
- [ ] 100 grams/3.5 oz
- [ ] Other: _____

Vegetable:
- [ ] Asparagus
- [ ] Beet Greens
- [ ] Cabbage
- [ ] Celery
- [ ] Chard
- [ ] Cucumber
- [ ] Fennel
- [ ] Lettuce
- [ ] Onions
- [ ] Radishes
- [ ] Spinach
- [ ] Tomatoes
- [ ] Other: _____
- [ ] Other: _____
- [ ] Other: _____

Fruit:
- [ ] Strawberries
- [ ] ½ Grapefruit
- [ ] Apple
- [ ] Orange
- [ ] Other: _____

Starch:
- [ ] Grissini
- [ ] Melba
- [ ] Other: _____

Other:
- [ ] TBS. Milk
- [ ] Juice of 1 Lemon
- [ ] Stevia
- [ ] Shirataki/Miracle Noodles
- [ ] Other: _____
- [ ] Other: _____
- [ ] Other: _____

Calories: _____ Calories: _____ Calories: _____ Calories: _____

DINNER Time : WAS AN ITEM EATEN AS A SNACK? WHICH? Time:

Protein:
- [ ] Chicken
- [ ] Beef
- [ ] Veal
- [ ] Shrimp
- [ ] Lobster
- [ ] White fish: _____
- [ ] Protein Shake
- [ ] Other: _____

Serving Size:
- [ ] 100 grams
- [ ] Other: _____

Vegetable:
- [ ] Asparagus
- [ ] Beet Greens
- [ ] Cabbage
- [ ] Celery
- [ ] Chard
- [ ] Cucumber
- [ ] Fennel
- [ ] Lettuce
- [ ] Onions
- [ ] Radishes
- [ ] Spinach
- [ ] Tomatoes
- [ ] Other: _____
- [ ] Other: _____
- [ ] Other: _____

Fruit:
- [ ] Strawberries
- [ ] ½ Grapefruit
- [ ] Apple
- [ ] Orange
- [ ] Other: _____

Starch:
- [ ] Grissini
- [ ] Melba
- [ ] Other: _____

Other:
- [ ] TBS. Milk
- [ ] Juice of 1 Lemon
- [ ] Stevia
- [ ] Shirataki/Miracle Noodles
- [ ] Other: _____
- [ ] Other: _____
- [ ] Other: _____

Calories: _____ Calories: _____ Calories: _____ Calories: _____

VLCD **14** (Date): _____

WEIGHT: _____

HCG DOSAGE: _____

HUNGER LEVEL: _____

BEDTIME/WAKE TIME: _____

HOURS SLEEP: _____

TOTAL CALORIES: _____

SUPPLEMENTS: _____

☐ Multivitamin ☐ B12 Shot ☐ Lipo Shot

FELLOW HCGER TIP:

hCG Coffee Dessert

100 grams fat free cottage cheese mixed with a dollop of fat free greek yogurt, stevia, and 1-2 tsp. instant coffee.

Note: If you do this, the cottage cheese would replace 1 meat protein serving.

INJECTION LOCATION   TIME: _____

☐ Belly ☐ Deltoid ☐ Thigh ☐ Other: _____

DROPS / PELLETS DOSE TIMING

1st Dose: _____   2nd Dose: _____
3rd Dose: _____   4th Dose: _____

PERSONAL NOTES

....

....

....

....

....

....

....

LIQUIDS:

4 LITERS	
3.5 LITERS	
3 LITERS	
2.5 LITERS	
2 LITERS	
1.5 LITERS	
1 LITER	
.5 LITERS	

128 oz = 1 GALLON	
120 oz	
112 oz	
104 oz	
96 oz = 3 QUARTS	
88 oz	
80 oz	
72 oz	
64 oz = 2 QUARTS	
56 oz	
48 oz	
40 oz	
32 oz = 1 QUART	
24 oz	
16 oz	
8 oz = 1 CUP	

BREAKFAST   Time : _____

☐ None ☐ Fruit: _____   ☐ Protein: _____   Calories: _____

Serving Size: _____   Serving Size: _____

LUNCH Time :   WAS AN ITEM EATEN AS A SNACK? WHICH?   Time:

Protein:
- [ ] Chicken breast
- [ ] Beef
- [ ] Veal
- [ ] Shrimp
- [ ] Lobster
- [ ] White fish: _____
- [ ] Protein Shake
- [ ] Other: _____

Serving Size:
- [ ] 100 grams/3.5 oz
- [ ] Other: _____

Vegetable:
- [ ] Asparagus
- [ ] Beet Greens
- [ ] Cabbage
- [ ] Celery
- [ ] Chard
- [ ] Cucumber
- [ ] Fennel
- [ ] Lettuce
- [ ] Onions
- [ ] Radishes
- [ ] Spinach
- [ ] Tomatoes
- [ ] Other: _____
- [ ] Other: _____
- [ ] Other: _____

Fruit:
- [ ] Strawberries
- [ ] ½ Grapefruit
- [ ] Apple
- [ ] Orange
- [ ] Other: _____

Starch:
- [ ] Grissini
- [ ] Melba
- [ ] Other: _____

Other:
- [ ] TBS. Milk
- [ ] Juice of 1 Lemon
- [ ] Stevia
- [ ] Shirataki/Miracle Noodles
- [ ] Other: _____
- [ ] Other: _____
- [ ] Other: _____

Calories: _____ Calories: _____ Calories: _____ Calories: _____

DINNER Time :   WAS AN ITEM EATEN AS A SNACK? WHICH?   Time:

Protein:
- [ ] Chicken
- [ ] Beef
- [ ] Veal
- [ ] Shrimp
- [ ] Lobster
- [ ] White fish: _____
- [ ] Protein Shake
- [ ] Other: _____

Serving Size:
- [ ] 100 grams
- [ ] Other: _____

Vegetable:
- [ ] Asparagus
- [ ] Beet Greens
- [ ] Cabbage
- [ ] Celery
- [ ] Chard
- [ ] Cucumber
- [ ] Fennel
- [ ] Lettuce
- [ ] Onions
- [ ] Radishes
- [ ] Spinach
- [ ] Tomatoes
- [ ] Other: _____
- [ ] Other: _____
- [ ] Other: _____

Fruit:
- [ ] Strawberries
- [ ] ½ Grapefruit
- [ ] Apple
- [ ] Orange
- [ ] Other: _____

Starch:
- [ ] Grissini
- [ ] Melba
- [ ] Other: _____

Other:
- [ ] TBS. Milk
- [ ] Juice of 1 Lemon
- [ ] Stevia
- [ ] Shirataki/Miracle Noodles
- [ ] Other: _____
- [ ] Other: _____
- [ ] Other: _____

Calories: _____ Calories: _____ Calories: _____ Calories: _____

Reflections ON WEEK 2

REMEMBER, THIS IS NOT JUST ABOUT LOSING WEIGHT. IT'S ABOUT CHANGING YOUR WHOLE MINDSET ABOUT FOOD AND YOUR BODY.

YOU ARE BREAKING OLD PATTERNS RIGHT NOW. YOU ARE CREATING NEW PATTERNS. TRY NOT TO FOCUS YOUR PROGESS SOLELY ON WEIGHT LOSS.

SO WITH THAT IN MIND, HOW DID THIS WEEK GO?

What are you proud of? Why are you proud of it? What did you struggle with? What would you like to work on changing? What specific logical ways can you think of to make those adjustments? Or maybe you're just burned out at the moment - it's okay to just make it a rant.

Prepping for PHASE 3 - ALREADY?

PHASE 3 NONCHALANCE = GAIN BACK WEIGHT.

I can honestly tell you that out of the many of emails I've received dealing specifically with **gaining back weight** that was lost with the hCG protocol, the number one cause that is shared with me for this happening is **not paying attention to Phase 3.**

Conversely, a do-over with subsequent strict attention to Phase 3 yielded much better, lasting results.

Your weight *will* be volatile at the start of Phase 3 and will go up easily if you don't have the knowledge and tools to know what to do or think it's not important.

This is not meant to scare you, but to iterate the importance of arming yourself with as much information for Phase 3 as you can, in advance, so you can have a plan when it arrives.

It might be easy to kind of freak out over Phase 3 a little, but as we've heard the saying go:

Worrying IS LIKE ROCKING IN A CHAIR. IT KEEPS YOU BUSY, BUT DOESN'T GET YOU ANYWHERE.

So let's NOT do that shall we?

INSTEAD, GET INFORMED and PLAN AHEAD. HOW?

I have 2 resources that can get you ready and prepared to face Phase 3 confidently. One is totally free, and the other costs a little $moola but gives you an exact roadmap and will help you learn to maintain like I have for 5 years now, without dieting over and over again anymore.

The P3 & P4 resources page on my site has QUITE a few articles and will help you both plan and troubleshoot.

The Phase 3 to Life program, gives you an EXACT roadmap to follow, and as you will see if you check out the program, many women have gone through it successfully now and stabilized and maintained their weight loss with ease. Yes I said it, ease. You don't have to be afraid of P3 if you have the right tools.

FREE BLOGPOSTS:
Simply: hcgchica.com/p3
hcgchica.com/p4

This is more general information but still gives you guidelines and tips for these phases.

STRUCTURED PHASE 3 PROGRAM:
the Phase 3 to Life Program
P3tolife.com

This is an exact program to follow in Phase 3 and beyond for long term maintenance.

UPDATE!

Hiya! Just wanted to let ya' know if you're finding this tracking tool helpful to your in your journey,

I NOW HAVE 2 OTHER VERSIONS OF THIS WORKBOOK.

1. THE DIGITAL WORKBOOK - a digital only file that once you purchase it, will be yours to use over and over forever and ever.

That's located at *hcgchica.com/workbook*.

----

2. RE-FILL PHYSICAL BOOK VERSION of the hCG diet workbook like this one.

You can **FIND IT ON AMAZON.COM** just by searching "hcg diet workbook" - the refill version is a bold YELLOW so you can't miss it. ;)

You can also learn more about the refill version on my blog at HCGCHICA.COM/RE-FILLWORKBOOK.

Why a refill version? It's a much thinner book, at a reduced cost, for your use on future rounds.

The refill version of the workbook takes out all the stuff you only need to have once (the diet instructions and the coaching etc- you'll always have that in this workbook) and leaves in all the stuff you'll need again for future rounds - the quick glance tracking and the daily tracking areas.

Week 5

"KNOWING TREES,
I understand the
meaning of patience.
Knowing grass,
I understand the
meaning of persistence. "

— Hal Borland

VLCD **15** (Date): _____

> Today is a new day. Hiding from your history only shackles you to it. WE CAN'T UNDO a single thing we have ever done, but WE CAN MAKE DECISIONS TODAY that propel us to the life we want and towards THE HEALING WE NEED.
> — Steve Maraboli

WEIGHT: _____

HCG DOSAGE: _____

HUNGER LEVEL: _____

BEDTIME/WAKE TIME: _____

HOURS SLEEP: _____

TOTAL CALORIES: _____

SUPPLEMENTS: _____

☐ Multivitamin ☐ B12 Shot ☐ Lipo Shot

INJECTION LOCATION   TIME: _____

☐ Belly ☐ Deltoid ☐ Thigh ☐ Other: _____

DROPS / PELLETS DOSE TIMING

1st Dose: _____   2nd Dose: _____

3rd Dose: _____   4th Dose: _____

PERSONAL NOTES

....

....

....

....

....

....

....

LIQUIDS:

4 LITERS	
3.5 LITERS	
3 LITERS	
2.5 LITERS	
2 LITERS	
1.5 LITERS	
1 LITER	
.5 LITERS	

128 oz = 1 GALLON	
120 oz	
112 oz	
104 oz	
96 oz = 3 QUARTS	
88 oz	
80 oz	
72 oz	
64 oz = 2 QUARTS	
56 oz	
48 oz	
40 oz	
32 oz = 1 QUART	
24 oz	
16 oz	
8 oz = 1 CUP	

BREAKFAST   Time :

☐ None ☐ Fruit: _____   ☐ Protein: _____   Calories: _____

Serving Size: _____   Serving Size: _____

LUNCH Time :   WAS AN ITEM EATEN AS A SNACK? WHICH?   Time:

Protein:
- [ ] Chicken breast
- [ ] Beef
- [ ] Veal
- [ ] Shrimp
- [ ] Lobster
- [ ] White fish: _____
- [ ] Protein Shake
- [ ] Other: _____

Serving Size:
- [ ] 100 grams/3.5 oz
- [ ] Other: _____

Calories: _____

Vegetable:
- [ ] Asparagus
- [ ] Beet Greens
- [ ] Cabbage
- [ ] Celery
- [ ] Chard
- [ ] Cucumber
- [ ] Fennel
- [ ] Lettuce
- [ ] Onions
- [ ] Radishes
- [ ] Spinach
- [ ] Tomatoes
- [ ] Other: _____
- [ ] Other: _____
- [ ] Other: _____

Calories: _____

Fruit:
- [ ] Strawberries
- [ ] ½ Grapefruit
- [ ] Apple
- [ ] Orange
- [ ] Other: _____

Starch:
- [ ] Grissini
- [ ] Melba
- [ ] Other: _____

Calories: _____

Other:
- [ ] TBS. Milk
- [ ] Juice of 1 Lemon
- [ ] Stevia
- [ ] Shirataki/Miracle Noodles
- [ ] Other: _____
- [ ] Other: _____
- [ ] Other: _____

Calories: _____

DINNER Time :   WAS AN ITEM EATEN AS A SNACK? WHICH?   Time:

Protein:
- [ ] Chicken
- [ ] Beef
- [ ] Veal
- [ ] Shrimp
- [ ] Lobster
- [ ] White fish: _____
- [ ] Protein Shake
- [ ] Other: _____

Serving Size:
- [ ] 100 grams
- [ ] Other: _____

Calories: _____

Vegetable:
- [ ] Asparagus
- [ ] Beet Greens
- [ ] Cabbage
- [ ] Celery
- [ ] Chard
- [ ] Cucumber
- [ ] Fennel
- [ ] Lettuce
- [ ] Onions
- [ ] Radishes
- [ ] Spinach
- [ ] Tomatoes
- [ ] Other: _____
- [ ] Other: _____
- [ ] Other: _____

Calories: _____

Fruit:
- [ ] Strawberries
- [ ] ½ Grapefruit
- [ ] Apple
- [ ] Orange
- [ ] Other: _____

Starch:
- [ ] Grissini
- [ ] Melba
- [ ] Other: _____

Calories: _____

Other:
- [ ] TBS. Milk
- [ ] Juice of 1 Lemon
- [ ] Stevia
- [ ] Shirataki/Miracle Noodles
- [ ] Other: _____
- [ ] Other: _____
- [ ] Other: _____

Calories: _____

HCGCHICA TIP:

You're Never Too Mature

Women in the 55-75 age bracket often email me, wondering if they are too, let's call it, mature, for this protocol to work for them. Let me just say this. The majority of my hCG success interviews are with women in this age bracket. Maturity has its benefits!

WEIGHT: _____

HCG DOSAGE: _____

HUNGER LEVEL: _____

BEDTIME/WAKE TIME: _____

HOURS SLEEP: _____

TOTAL CALORIES: _____

SUPPLEMENTS: _____

☐ Multivitamin   ☐ B12 Shot   ☐ Lipo Shot

INJECTION LOCATION   TIME: _____

☐ Belly   ☐ Deltoid   ☐ Thigh   ☐ Other: _____

DROPS / PELLETS DOSE TIMING

1st Dose: _____   2nd Dose: _____

3rd Dose: _____   4th Dose: _____

PERSONAL NOTES

....

....

....

....

....

....

....

LIQUIDS:

4 LITERS	
3.5 LITERS	
3 LITERS	
2.5 LITERS	
2 LITERS	
1.5 LITERS	
1 LITER	
.5 LITERS	

128 oz = 1 GALLON	
120 oz	
112 oz	
104 oz	
96 oz = 3 QUARTS	
88 oz	
80 oz	
72 oz	
64 oz = 2 QUARTS	
56 oz	
48 oz	
40 oz	
32 oz = 1 QUART	
24 oz	
16 oz	
8 oz = 1 CUP	

BREAKFAST   Time: _____

☐ None   ☐ Fruit: _____   ☐ Protein: _____   Calories: _____

Serving Size: _____   Serving Size: _____

LUNCH Time: WAS AN ITEM EATEN AS A SNACK? WHICH?   Time:

Protein:
- ☐ Chicken breast
- ☐ Beef
- ☐ Veal
- ☐ Shrimp
- ☐ Lobster
- ☐ White fish: _____
- ☐ Protein Shake
- ☐ Other: _____

Serving Size:
- ☐ 100 grams/3.5 oz
- ☐ Other: _____

Vegetable:
- ☐ Asparagus
- ☐ Beet Greens
- ☐ Cabbage
- ☐ Celery
- ☐ Chard
- ☐ Cucumber
- ☐ Fennel
- ☐ Lettuce
- ☐ Onions
- ☐ Radishes
- ☐ Spinach
- ☐ Tomatoes
- ☐ Other: _____
- ☐ Other: _____
- ☐ Other: _____

Fruit:
- ☐ Strawberries
- ☐ ½ Grapefruit
- ☐ Apple
- ☐ Orange
- ☐ Other: _____

Starch:
- ☐ Grissini
- ☐ Melba
- ☐ Other: _____

Other:
- ☐ TBS. Milk
- ☐ Juice of 1 Lemon
- ☐ Stevia
- ☐ Shirataki/Miracle Noodles
- ☐ Other: _____
- ☐ Other: _____
- ☐ Other: _____

Calories: _____   Calories: _____   Calories: _____   Calories: _____

DINNER Time: WAS AN ITEM EATEN AS A SNACK? WHICH?   Time:

Protein:
- ☐ Chicken
- ☐ Beef
- ☐ Veal
- ☐ Shrimp
- ☐ Lobster
- ☐ White fish: _____
- ☐ Protein Shake
- ☐ Other: _____

Serving Size:
- ☐ 100 grams
- ☐ Other: _____

Vegetable:
- ☐ Asparagus
- ☐ Beet Greens
- ☐ Cabbage
- ☐ Celery
- ☐ Chard
- ☐ Cucumber
- ☐ Fennel
- ☐ Lettuce
- ☐ Onions
- ☐ Radishes
- ☐ Spinach
- ☐ Tomatoes
- ☐ Other: _____
- ☐ Other: _____
- ☐ Other: _____

Fruit:
- ☐ Strawberries
- ☐ ½ Grapefruit
- ☐ Apple
- ☐ Orange
- ☐ Other: _____

Starch:
- ☐ Grissini
- ☐ Melba
- ☐ Other: _____

Other:
- ☐ TBS. Milk
- ☐ Juice of 1 Lemon
- ☐ Stevia
- ☐ Shirataki/Miracle Noodles
- ☐ Other: _____
- ☐ Other: _____
- ☐ Other: _____

Calories: _____   Calories: _____   Calories: _____   Calories: _____

FELLOW HCGER TIP:

Make it Fire Roasted

When it comes to canned tomatoes, the "fire roasted" kind have SO much more flavor than the regular kind.

Note: Be sure to check the ingredient label as some brands of canned tomatoes have added sugar.

WEIGHT: _____

HCG DOSAGE: _____

HUNGER LEVEL: _____

BEDTIME/WAKE TIME: _____

HOURS SLEEP: _____

TOTAL CALORIES: _____

SUPPLEMENTS: _____

☐ Multivitamin   ☐ B12 Shot   ☐ Lipo Shot

INJECTION LOCATION   TIME: _____

☐ Belly   ☐ Deltoid   ☐ Thigh   ☐ Other: _____

DROPS / PELLETS DOSE TIMING

1st Dose: _____   2nd Dose: _____

3rd Dose: _____   4th Dose: _____

PERSONAL NOTES

....

....

....

....

....

....

....

LIQUIDS:

4 LITERS	128 oz = 1 GALLON
3.5 LITERS	120 oz
3 LITERS	112 oz
2.5 LITERS	104 oz
2 LITERS	96 oz = 3 QUARTS
1.5 LITERS	88 oz
1 LITER	80 oz
.5 LITERS	72 oz
	64 oz = 2 QUARTS
	56 oz
	48 oz
	40 oz
	32 oz = 1 QUART
	24 oz
	16 oz
	8 oz = 1 CUP

BREAKFAST   Time :

☐ None   ☐ Fruit: _____   ☐ Protein: _____   Calories: _____

Serving Size: _____   Serving Size: _____

LUNCH Time : .... WAS AN ITEM EATEN AS A SNACK? WHICH?   Time:

Protein:
- ☐ Chicken breast
- ☐ Beef
- ☐ Veal
- ☐ Shrimp
- ☐ Lobster
- ☐ White fish: _____
- ☐ Protein Shake
- ☐ Other: _____

Serving Size:
- ☐ 100 grams/3.5 oz
- ☐ Other: _____

Vegetable:
- ☐ Asparagus
- ☐ Beet Greens
- ☐ Cabbage
- ☐ Celery
- ☐ Chard
- ☐ Cucumber
- ☐ Fennel
- ☐ Lettuce
- ☐ Onions
- ☐ Radishes
- ☐ Spinach
- ☐ Tomatoes
- ☐ Other: _____
- ☐ Other: _____
- ☐ Other: _____

Fruit:
- ☐ Strawberries
- ☐ ½ Grapefruit
- ☐ Apple
- ☐ Orange
- ☐ Other: _____

Starch:
- ☐ Grissini
- ☐ Melba
- ☐ Other: _____

Other:
- ☐ TBS. Milk
- ☐ Juice of 1 Lemon
- ☐ Stevia
- ☐ Shirataki/Miracle Noodles
- ☐ Other: _____
- ☐ Other: _____
- ☐ Other: _____

Calories: _____   Calories: _____   Calories: _____   Calories: _____

DINNER Time : .... WAS AN ITEM EATEN AS A SNACK? WHICH?   Time:

Protein:
- ☐ Chicken
- ☐ Beef
- ☐ Veal
- ☐ Shrimp
- ☐ Lobster
- ☐ White fish: _____
- ☐ Protein Shake
- ☐ Other: _____

Serving Size:
- ☐ 100 grams
- ☐ Other: _____

Vegetable:
- ☐ Asparagus
- ☐ Beet Greens
- ☐ Cabbage
- ☐ Celery
- ☐ Chard
- ☐ Cucumber
- ☐ Fennel
- ☐ Lettuce
- ☐ Onions
- ☐ Radishes
- ☐ Spinach
- ☐ Tomatoes
- ☐ Other: _____
- ☐ Other: _____
- ☐ Other: _____

Fruit:
- ☐ Strawberries
- ☐ ½ Grapefruit
- ☐ Apple
- ☐ Orange
- ☐ Other: _____

Starch:
- ☐ Grissini
- ☐ Melba
- ☐ Other: _____

Other:
- ☐ TBS. Milk
- ☐ Juice of 1 Lemon
- ☐ Stevia
- ☐ Shirataki/Miracle Noodles
- ☐ Other: _____
- ☐ Other: _____
- ☐ Other: _____

Calories: _____   Calories: _____   Calories: _____   Calories: _____

VLCD 18 (Date): _____

WEIGHT: _____

HCG DOSAGE: _____

HUNGER LEVEL: _____

BEDTIME/WAKE TIME: _____

HOURS SLEEP: _____

TOTAL CALORIES: _____

SUPPLEMENTS: _____

☐ Multivitamin ☐ B12 Shot ☐ Lipo Shot

> When we complain we are saying we do not have the POWER TO MAKE A DIFFERENCE in the situation and *we make ourselves small*... we become part of the problem instead of the solution! TAKE ACTION to make the situation better & live bigger!
> – Jefroy Hanson

INJECTION LOCATION   TIME: _____

☐ Belly ☐ Deltoid ☐ Thigh ☐ Other: _____

DROPS / PELLETS DOSE TIMING

1st Dose: _____   2nd Dose: _____

3rd Dose: _____   4th Dose: _____

PERSONAL NOTES

....

_____

_____

_____

_____

_____

_____

_____

LIQUIDS:

4 LITERS	128 oz = 1 GALLON
3.5 LITERS	120 oz
3 LITERS	112 oz
2.5 LITERS	104 oz
2 LITERS	96 oz = 3 QUARTS
1.5 LITERS	88 oz
1 LITER	80 oz
.5 LITERS	72 oz
	64 oz = 2 QUARTS
	56 oz
	48 oz
	40 oz
	32 oz = 1 QUART
	24 oz
	16 oz
	8 oz = 1 CUP

BREAKFAST   Time:

....

☐ None ☐ Fruit: _____ ☐ Protein: _____ Calories: _____

Serving Size: _____   Serving Size: _____

LUNCH Time : _____   WAS AN ITEM EATEN AS A SNACK? WHICH?   Time: _____

Protein:
- [ ] Chicken breast
- [ ] Beef
- [ ] Veal
- [ ] Shrimp
- [ ] Lobster
- [ ] White fish: _____
- [ ] Protein Shake
- [ ] Other: _____

Serving Size:
- [ ] 100 grams/3.5 oz
- [ ] Other: _____

Vegetable:
- [ ] Asparagus
- [ ] Beet Greens
- [ ] Cabbage
- [ ] Celery
- [ ] Chard
- [ ] Cucumber
- [ ] Fennel
- [ ] Lettuce
- [ ] Onions
- [ ] Radishes
- [ ] Spinach
- [ ] Tomatoes
- [ ] Other: _____
- [ ] Other: _____
- [ ] Other: _____

Fruit:
- [ ] Strawberries
- [ ] ½ Grapefruit
- [ ] Apple
- [ ] Orange
- [ ] Other: _____

Starch:
- [ ] Grissini
- [ ] Melba
- [ ] Other: _____

Other:
- [ ] TBS. Milk
- [ ] Juice of 1 Lemon
- [ ] Stevia
- [ ] Shirataki/Miracle Noodles
- [ ] Other: _____
- [ ] Other: _____
- [ ] Other: _____

Calories: _____   Calories: _____   Calories: _____   Calories: _____

DINNER Time : _____   WAS AN ITEM EATEN AS A SNACK? WHICH?   Time: _____

Protein:
- [ ] Chicken
- [ ] Beef
- [ ] Veal
- [ ] Shrimp
- [ ] Lobster
- [ ] White fish: _____
- [ ] Protein Shake
- [ ] Other: _____

Serving Size:
- [ ] 100 grams
- [ ] Other: _____

Vegetable:
- [ ] Asparagus
- [ ] Beet Greens
- [ ] Cabbage
- [ ] Celery
- [ ] Chard
- [ ] Cucumber
- [ ] Fennel
- [ ] Lettuce
- [ ] Onions
- [ ] Radishes
- [ ] Spinach
- [ ] Tomatoes
- [ ] Other: _____
- [ ] Other: _____
- [ ] Other: _____

Fruit:
- [ ] Strawberries
- [ ] ½ Grapefruit
- [ ] Apple
- [ ] Orange
- [ ] Other: _____

Starch:
- [ ] Grissini
- [ ] Melba
- [ ] Other: _____

Other:
- [ ] TBS. Milk
- [ ] Juice of 1 Lemon
- [ ] Stevia
- [ ] Shirataki/Miracle Noodles
- [ ] Other: _____
- [ ] Other: _____
- [ ] Other: _____

Calories: _____   Calories: _____   Calories: _____   Calories: _____

VLCD 19 (Date): _____

WEIGHT: _____

HCG DOSAGE: _____

HUNGER LEVEL: _____

BEDTIME/WAKE TIME: _____

HOURS SLEEP: _____

TOTAL CALORIES: _____

SUPPLEMENTS: _____

☐ Multivitamin   ☐ B12 Shot   ☐ Lipo Shot

FELLOW HCGER TIP:

When You Need Quick

Keep a container in the fridge with chopped hCG veggies so you can quickly prepare a meal when in a hurry.

INJECTION LOCATION   TIME: _____

☐ Belly   ☐ Deltoid   ☐ Thigh   ☐ Other: _____

DROPS / PELLETS DOSE TIMING

1st Dose: _____   2nd Dose: _____

3rd Dose: _____   4th Dose: _____

PERSONAL NOTES

....
....
....
....
....
....
....

LIQUIDS:

4	LITERS	
3.5	LITERS	
3	LITERS	
2.5	LITERS	
2	LITERS	
1.5	LITERS	
1	LITER	
.5	LITERS	

128 oz	= 1 GALLON
120 oz	
112 oz	
104 oz	
96 oz	= 3 QUARTS
88 oz	
80 oz	
72 oz	
64 oz	= 2 QUARTS
56 oz	
48 oz	
40 oz	
32 oz	= 1 QUART
24 oz	
16 oz	
8 oz	= 1 CUP

BREAKFAST   Time :

☐ None   ☐ Fruit: _____   ☐ Protein: _____   Calories: _____

Serving Size: _____   Serving Size: _____

LUNCH Time: _____

Protein:
- [ ] Chicken breast
- [ ] Beef
- [ ] Veal
- [ ] Shrimp
- [ ] Lobster
- [ ] White fish: _____
- [ ] Protein Shake
- [ ] Other: _____

Serving Size:
- [ ] 100 grams/3.5 oz
- [ ] Other: _____

Vegetable:
- [ ] Asparagus
- [ ] Beet Greens
- [ ] Cabbage
- [ ] Celery
- [ ] Chard
- [ ] Cucumber
- [ ] Fennel
- [ ] Lettuce
- [ ] Onions
- [ ] Radishes
- [ ] Spinach
- [ ] Tomatoes
- [ ] Other: _____
- [ ] Other: _____
- [ ] Other: _____

Fruit:
- [ ] Strawberries
- [ ] ½ Grapefruit
- [ ] Apple
- [ ] Orange
- [ ] Other: _____

Starch:
- [ ] Grissini
- [ ] Melba
- [ ] Other: _____

Other:
- [ ] TBS. Milk
- [ ] Juice of 1 Lemon
- [ ] Stevia
- [ ] Shirataki/Miracle Noodles
- [ ] Other: _____
- [ ] Other: _____
- [ ] Other: _____

Calories: _____   Calories: _____   Calories: _____   Calories: _____

DINNER Time: _____

Protein:
- [ ] Chicken
- [ ] Beef
- [ ] Veal
- [ ] Shrimp
- [ ] Lobster
- [ ] White fish: _____
- [ ] Protein Shake
- [ ] Other: _____

Serving Size:
- [ ] 100 grams
- [ ] Other: _____

Vegetable:
- [ ] Asparagus
- [ ] Beet Greens
- [ ] Cabbage
- [ ] Celery
- [ ] Chard
- [ ] Cucumber
- [ ] Fennel
- [ ] Lettuce
- [ ] Onions
- [ ] Radishes
- [ ] Spinach
- [ ] Tomatoes
- [ ] Other: _____
- [ ] Other: _____
- [ ] Other: _____

Fruit:
- [ ] Strawberries
- [ ] ½ Grapefruit
- [ ] Apple
- [ ] Orange
- [ ] Other: _____

Starch:
- [ ] Grissini
- [ ] Melba
- [ ] Other: _____

Other:
- [ ] TBS. Milk
- [ ] Juice of 1 Lemon
- [ ] Stevia
- [ ] Shirataki/Miracle Noodles
- [ ] Other: _____
- [ ] Other: _____
- [ ] Other: _____

Calories: _____   Calories: _____   Calories: _____   Calories: _____

VLCD **20** (Date): _____

WEIGHT: _____

HCG DOSAGE: _____

HUNGER LEVEL: _____

BEDTIME/WAKE TIME: _____

HOURS SLEEP: _____

TOTAL CALORIES: _____

SUPPLEMENTS: _____

☐ Multivitamin   ☐ B12 Shot   ☐ Lipo Shot

> *Courage*
> doesn't always roar.
> Sometimes courage is
> THE QUIET VOICE
> at the end of the day saying,
> 'I will try again tomorrow.
>
> *- Mary Anne Radmacher*

INJECTION LOCATION   TIME: _____

☐ Belly   ☐ Deltoid   ☐ Thigh   ☐ Other: _____

DROPS / PELLETS DOSE TIMING

1st Dose: _____   2nd Dose: _____

3rd Dose: _____   4th Dose: _____

PERSONAL NOTES

....

....

....

....

....

....

....

LIQUIDS:

4 LITERS	128 oz = 1 GALLON
3.5 LITERS	120 oz
3 LITERS	112 oz
2.5 LITERS	104 oz
2 LITERS	96 oz = 3 QUARTS
1.5 LITERS	88 oz
1 LITER	80 oz
.5 LITERS	72 oz
	64 oz = 2 QUARTS
	56 oz
	48 oz
	40 oz
	32 oz = 1 QUART
	24 oz
	16 oz
	8 oz = 1 CUP

BREAKFAST   Time :

☐ None   ☐ Fruit: _____   ☐ Protein: _____   Calories: _____

Serving Size: _____   Serving Size: _____

LUNCH Time :   WAS AN ITEM EATEN AS A SNACK? WHICH?   Time:

Protein:

- [ ] Chicken breast
- [ ] Beef
- [ ] Veal
- [ ] Shrimp
- [ ] Lobster
- [ ] White fish: _____
- [ ] Protein Shake
- [ ] Other: _____

Serving Size:
- [ ] 100 grams/3.5 oz
- [ ] Other: _____

Vegetable:

- [ ] Asparagus
- [ ] Beet Greens
- [ ] Cabbage
- [ ] Celery
- [ ] Chard
- [ ] Cucumber
- [ ] Fennel
- [ ] Lettuce
- [ ] Onions
- [ ] Radishes
- [ ] Spinach
- [ ] Tomatoes
- [ ] Other: _____
- [ ] Other: _____
- [ ] Other: _____

Fruit:

- [ ] Strawberries
- [ ] ½ Grapefruit
- [ ] Apple
- [ ] Orange
- [ ] Other: _____

Starch:

- [ ] Grissini
- [ ] Melba
- [ ] Other: _____

Other:

- [ ] TBS. Milk
- [ ] Juice of 1 Lemon
- [ ] Stevia
- [ ] Shirataki/Miracle Noodles
- [ ] Other: _____
- [ ] Other: _____
- [ ] Other: _____

Calories: _____   Calories: _____   Calories: _____   Calories: _____

DINNER Time :   WAS AN ITEM EATEN AS A SNACK? WHICH?   Time:

Protein:

- [ ] Chicken
- [ ] Beef
- [ ] Veal
- [ ] Shrimp
- [ ] Lobster
- [ ] White fish: _____
- [ ] Protein Shake
- [ ] Other: _____

Serving Size:
- [ ] 100 grams
- [ ] Other: _____

Vegetable:

- [ ] Asparagus
- [ ] Beet Greens
- [ ] Cabbage
- [ ] Celery
- [ ] Chard
- [ ] Cucumber
- [ ] Fennel
- [ ] Lettuce
- [ ] Onions
- [ ] Radishes
- [ ] Spinach
- [ ] Tomatoes
- [ ] Other: _____
- [ ] Other: _____
- [ ] Other: _____

Fruit:

- [ ] Strawberries
- [ ] ½ Grapefruit
- [ ] Apple
- [ ] Orange
- [ ] Other: _____

Starch:

- [ ] Grissini
- [ ] Melba
- [ ] Other: _____

Other:

- [ ] TBS. Milk
- [ ] Juice of 1 Lemon
- [ ] Stevia
- [ ] Shirataki/Miracle Noodles
- [ ] Other: _____
- [ ] Other: _____
- [ ] Other: _____

Calories: _____   Calories: _____   Calories: _____   Calories: _____

VLCD 21 (Date): _____

WEIGHT: _____

HCG DOSAGE: _____

HUNGER LEVEL: _____

BEDTIME/WAKE TIME: _____

HOURS SLEEP: _____

TOTAL CALORIES: _____

SUPPLEMENTS: _____

☐ Multivitamin   ☐ B12 Shot   ☐ Lipo Shot

INJECTION LOCATION   TIME: _____

☐ Belly   ☐ Deltoid   ☐ Thigh   ☐ Other: _____

DROPS / PELLETS DOSE TIMING

1st Dose: _____   2nd Dose: _____
3rd Dose: _____   4th Dose: _____

PERSONAL NOTES

....

....

....

....

....

....

....

....

LIQUIDS:

4	LITERS	
3.5	LITERS	
3	LITERS	
2.5	LITERS	
2	LITERS	
1.5	LITERS	
1	LITER	
.5	LITERS	

128 oz	= 1 GALLON
120 oz	
112 oz	
104 oz	
96 oz	= 3 QUARTS
88 oz	
80 oz	
72 oz	
64 oz	= 2 QUARTS
56 oz	
48 oz	
40 oz	
32 oz	= 1 QUART
24 oz	
16 oz	
8 oz	= 1 CUP

BREAKFAST   Time :

☐ None   ☐ Fruit: _____   ☐ Protein: _____   *Calories:* _____

Serving Size: _____   *Serving Size:* _____

LUNCH Time: WAS AN ITEM EATEN AS A SNACK? WHICH?   Time:

Protein:
- [ ] Chicken breast
- [ ] Beef
- [ ] Veal
- [ ] Shrimp
- [ ] Lobster
- [ ] White fish: _____
- [ ] Protein Shake
- [ ] Other: _____

Serving Size:
- [ ] 100 grams/3.5 oz
- [ ] Other: _____

Vegetable:
- [ ] Asparagus
- [ ] Beet Greens
- [ ] Cabbage
- [ ] Celery
- [ ] Chard
- [ ] Cucumber
- [ ] Fennel
- [ ] Lettuce
- [ ] Onions
- [ ] Radishes
- [ ] Spinach
- [ ] Tomatoes
- [ ] Other: _____
- [ ] Other: _____
- [ ] Other: _____

Fruit:
- [ ] Strawberries
- [ ] ½ Grapefruit
- [ ] Apple
- [ ] Orange
- [ ] Other: _____

Starch:
- [ ] Grissini
- [ ] Melba
- [ ] Other: _____

Other:
- [ ] TBS. Milk
- [ ] Juice of 1 Lemon
- [ ] Stevia
- [ ] Shirataki/Miracle Noodles
- [ ] Other: _____
- [ ] Other: _____
- [ ] Other: _____

Calories: _____   Calories: _____   Calories: _____   Calories: _____

DINNER Time: WAS AN ITEM EATEN AS A SNACK? WHICH?   Time:

Protein:
- [ ] Chicken
- [ ] Beef
- [ ] Veal
- [ ] Shrimp
- [ ] Lobster
- [ ] White fish: _____
- [ ] Protein Shake
- [ ] Other: _____

Serving Size:
- [ ] 100 grams
- [ ] Other: _____

Vegetable:
- [ ] Asparagus
- [ ] Beet Greens
- [ ] Cabbage
- [ ] Celery
- [ ] Chard
- [ ] Cucumber
- [ ] Fennel
- [ ] Lettuce
- [ ] Onions
- [ ] Radishes
- [ ] Spinach
- [ ] Tomatoes
- [ ] Other: _____
- [ ] Other: _____
- [ ] Other: _____

Fruit:
- [ ] Strawberries
- [ ] ½ Grapefruit
- [ ] Apple
- [ ] Orange
- [ ] Other: _____

Starch:
- [ ] Grissini
- [ ] Melba
- [ ] Other: _____

Other:
- [ ] TBS. Milk
- [ ] Juice of 1 Lemon
- [ ] Stevia
- [ ] Shirataki/Miracle Noodles
- [ ] Other: _____
- [ ] Other: _____
- [ ] Other: _____

Calories: _____   Calories: _____   Calories: _____   Calories: _____

Reflections ON WEEK 3

REMEMBER, THIS IS NOT JUST ABOUT LOSING WEIGHT. IT'S ABOUT CHANGING YOUR WHOLE MINDSET ABOUT FOOD AND YOUR BODY.

YOU ARE BREAKING OLD PATTERNS RIGHT NOW. YOU ARE CREATING NEW PATTERNS. TRY NOT TO FOCUS YOUR PROGESS SOLELY ON WEIGHT LOSS.

SO WITH THAT IN MIND, HOW DID THIS WEEK GO?

What are you proud of? Why are you proud of it? What did you struggle with? What would you like to work on changing? What specific logical ways can you think of to make those adjustments? Or maybe you're just burned out at the moment - it's okay to just make it a rant.

....
....
....
....
....
....
....
....
....
....
....
....
....
....
....
....

Week 4

"IT MAY TAKE A LITTLE TIME to get where you want to be, but if you pause and think for a moment, you will notice that you are no longer where you were. Do not stop - keep going."

— Rodolfo Costa

VLCD **22** (Date): _____

> And the *day came* when the **RISK TO REMAIN** tight in a bud was more painful than the **RISK** it took to *blossom.*
>
> *- Anais Nin*

WEIGHT: _____

HCG DOSAGE: _____

HUNGER LEVEL: _____

BEDTIME/WAKE TIME: _____

HOURS SLEEP: _____

TOTAL CALORIES: _____

SUPPLEMENTS: _____

☐ Multivitamin   ☐ B12 Shot   ☐ Lipo Shot

INJECTION LOCATION   TIME: _____

☐ Belly   ☐ Deltoid   ☐ Thigh   ☐ Other: _____

DROPS / PELLETS DOSE TIMING

1st Dose: _____   2nd Dose: _____

3rd Dose: _____   4th Dose: _____

PERSONAL NOTES

....

....

....

....

....

....

....

LIQUIDS:

4 LITERS	128 oz = 1 GALLON
3.5 LITERS	120 oz
3 LITERS	112 oz
2.5 LITERS	104 oz
2 LITERS	96 oz = 3 QUARTS
1.5 LITERS	88 oz
1 LITER	80 oz
.5 LITERS	72 oz
	64 oz = 2 QUARTS
	56 oz
	48 oz
	40 oz
	32 oz = 1 QUART
	24 oz
	16 oz
	8 oz = 1 CUP

BREAKFAST   Time : _____

☐ None   ☐ Fruit: _____   ☐ Protein: _____   Calories: _____

Serving Size: _____   Serving Size: _____

LUNCH Time :

Time:

Protein:
- [ ] Chicken breast
- [ ] Beef
- [ ] Veal
- [ ] Shrimp
- [ ] Lobster
- [ ] White fish: _____
- [ ] Protein Shake
- [ ] Other: _____

Serving Size:
- [ ] 100 grams/3.5 oz
- [ ] Other: _____

Calories: _____

Vegetable:
- [ ] Asparagus
- [ ] Beet Greens
- [ ] Cabbage
- [ ] Celery
- [ ] Chard
- [ ] Cucumber
- [ ] Fennel
- [ ] Lettuce
- [ ] Onions
- [ ] Radishes
- [ ] Spinach
- [ ] Tomatoes
- [ ] Other: _____
- [ ] Other: _____
- [ ] Other: _____

Calories: _____

Fruit:
- [ ] Strawberries
- [ ] ½ Grapefruit
- [ ] Apple
- [ ] Orange
- [ ] Other: _____

Starch:
- [ ] Grissini
- [ ] Melba
- [ ] Other: _____

Calories: _____

Other:
- [ ] TBS. Milk
- [ ] Juice of 1 Lemon
- [ ] Stevia
- [ ] Shirataki/Miracle Noodles
- [ ] Other: _____
- [ ] Other: _____
- [ ] Other: _____

Calories: _____

DINNER Time :

WAS AN ITEM EATEN AS A SNACK? WHICH? Time:

Protein:
- [ ] Chicken
- [ ] Beef
- [ ] Veal
- [ ] Shrimp
- [ ] Lobster
- [ ] White fish: _____
- [ ] Protein Shake
- [ ] Other: _____

Serving Size:
- [ ] 100 grams
- [ ] Other: _____

Calories: _____

Vegetable:
- [ ] Asparagus
- [ ] Beet Greens
- [ ] Cabbage
- [ ] Celery
- [ ] Chard
- [ ] Cucumber
- [ ] Fennel
- [ ] Lettuce
- [ ] Onions
- [ ] Radishes
- [ ] Spinach
- [ ] Tomatoes
- [ ] Other: _____
- [ ] Other: _____
- [ ] Other: _____

Calories: _____

Fruit:
- [ ] Strawberries
- [ ] ½ Grapefruit
- [ ] Apple
- [ ] Orange
- [ ] Other: _____

Starch:
- [ ] Grissini
- [ ] Melba
- [ ] Other: _____

Calories: _____

Other:
- [ ] TBS. Milk
- [ ] Juice of 1 Lemon
- [ ] Stevia
- [ ] Shirataki/Miracle Noodles
- [ ] Other: _____
- [ ] Other: _____
- [ ] Other: _____

Calories: _____

VLCD **23** (Date): _____

WEIGHT: _____

HCG DOSAGE: _____

HUNGER LEVEL: _____

BEDTIME/WAKE TIME: _____

HOURS SLEEP: _____

TOTAL CALORIES: _____

SUPPLEMENTS: _____

☐ Multivitamin   ☐ B12 Shot   ☐ Lipo Shot

INJECTION LOCATION   TIME: _____

☐ Belly   ☐ Deltoid   ☐ Thigh   ☐ Other: _____

DROPS / PELLETS DOSE TIMING

1st Dose: _____   2nd Dose: _____

3rd Dose: _____   4th Dose: _____

PERSONAL NOTES

....

....

....

....

....

....

....

LIQUIDS:

4 LITERS	128 oz = 1 GALLON
3.5 LITERS	120 oz
3 LITERS	112 oz
2.5 LITERS	104 oz
2 LITERS	96 oz = 3 QUARTS
1.5 LITERS	88 oz
1 LITER	80 oz
.5 LITERS	72 oz
	64 oz = 2 QUARTS
	56 oz
	48 oz
	40 oz
	32 oz = 1 QUART
	24 oz
	16 oz
	8 oz = 1 CUP

BREAKFAST   Time :

☐ None   ☐ Fruit: _____   ☐ Protein: _____   Calories: _____

Serving Size: _____   Serving Size: _____

LUNCH Time:

Protein:
- [ ] Chicken breast
- [ ] Beef
- [ ] Veal
- [ ] Shrimp
- [ ] Lobster
- [ ] White fish: _____
- [ ] Protein Shake
- [ ] Other: _____

Serving Size:
- [ ] 100 grams/3.5 oz
- [ ] Other: _____

Calories: _____

Vegetable:
- [ ] Asparagus
- [ ] Beet Greens
- [ ] Cabbage
- [ ] Celery
- [ ] Chard
- [ ] Cucumber
- [ ] Fennel
- [ ] Lettuce
- [ ] Onions
- [ ] Radishes
- [ ] Spinach
- [ ] Tomatoes
- [ ] Other: _____
- [ ] Other: _____
- [ ] Other: _____

Calories: _____

Fruit:
- [ ] Strawberries
- [ ] ½ Grapefruit
- [ ] Apple
- [ ] Orange
- [ ] Other: _____

Starch:
- [ ] Grissini
- [ ] Melba
- [ ] Other: _____

Calories: _____

Other:
- [ ] TBS. Milk
- [ ] Juice of 1 Lemon
- [ ] Stevia
- [ ] Shirataki/Miracle Noodles
- [ ] Other: _____
- [ ] Other: _____
- [ ] Other: _____

Calories: _____

DINNER Time:

Protein:
- [ ] Chicken
- [ ] Beef
- [ ] Veal
- [ ] Shrimp
- [ ] Lobster
- [ ] White fish: _____
- [ ] Protein Shake
- [ ] Other: _____

Serving Size:
- [ ] 100 grams
- [ ] Other: _____

Calories: _____

Vegetable:
- [ ] Asparagus
- [ ] Beet Greens
- [ ] Cabbage
- [ ] Celery
- [ ] Chard
- [ ] Cucumber
- [ ] Fennel
- [ ] Lettuce
- [ ] Onions
- [ ] Radishes
- [ ] Spinach
- [ ] Tomatoes
- [ ] Other: _____
- [ ] Other: _____
- [ ] Other: _____

Calories: _____

Fruit:
- [ ] Strawberries
- [ ] ½ Grapefruit
- [ ] Apple
- [ ] Orange
- [ ] Other: _____

Starch:
- [ ] Grissini
- [ ] Melba
- [ ] Other: _____

Calories: _____

Other:
- [ ] TBS. Milk
- [ ] Juice of 1 Lemon
- [ ] Stevia
- [ ] Shirataki/Miracle Noodles
- [ ] Other: _____
- [ ] Other: _____
- [ ] Other: _____

Calories: _____

VLCD **24** (Date): _____

WEIGHT: _____

HCG DOSAGE: _____

HUNGER LEVEL: _____

BEDTIME/WAKE TIME: _____

HOURS SLEEP: _____

TOTAL CALORIES: _____

SUPPLEMENTS: _____

☐ Multivitamin ☐ B12 Shot ☐ Lipo Shot

> Most **GOOD DECISIONS**
> that a person makes
> are a result of *reflection*
> and the **WILL TO CHANGE.**
>
> - *Innocent Mwatsikesimbe*

INJECTION LOCATION   TIME: _____

☐ Belly ☐ Deltoid ☐ Thigh ☐ Other: _____

DROPS / PELLETS DOSE TIMING

1st Dose: _____ 2nd Dose: _____

3rd Dose: _____ 4th Dose: _____

PERSONAL NOTES

....
....
....
....
....
....
....
....

LIQUIDS:

4 LITERS		128 oz = 1 GALLON
3.5 LITERS		120 oz
3 LITERS		112 oz
2.5 LITERS		104 oz
2 LITERS		96 oz = 3 QUARTS
1.5 LITERS		88 oz
1 LITER		80 oz
.5 LITERS		72 oz
		64 oz = 2 QUARTS
		56 oz
		48 oz
		40 oz
		32 oz = 1 QUART
		24 oz
		16 oz
		8 oz = 1 CUP

BREAKFAST   Time :

☐ None ☐ Fruit: _____   ☐ Protein: _____   *Calories:* _____

Serving Size: _____   Serving Size: _____

LUNCH Time :   WAS AN ITEM EATEN AS A SNACK? WHICH?   Time:

Protein:
- [ ] Chicken breast
- [ ] Beef
- [ ] Veal
- [ ] Shrimp
- [ ] Lobster
- [ ] White fish: _____
- [ ] Protein Shake
- [ ] Other: _____

Serving Size:
- [ ] 100 grams/3.5 oz
- [ ] Other: _____

Calories: _____

Vegetable:
- [ ] Asparagus
- [ ] Beet Greens
- [ ] Cabbage
- [ ] Celery
- [ ] Chard
- [ ] Cucumber
- [ ] Fennel
- [ ] Lettuce
- [ ] Onions
- [ ] Radishes
- [ ] Spinach
- [ ] Tomatoes
- [ ] Other: _____
- [ ] Other: _____
- [ ] Other: _____

Calories: _____

Fruit:
- [ ] Strawberries
- [ ] ½ Grapefruit
- [ ] Apple
- [ ] Orange
- [ ] Other: _____

Starch:
- [ ] Grissini
- [ ] Melba
- [ ] Other: _____

Calories: _____

Other:
- [ ] TBS. Milk
- [ ] Juice of 1 Lemon
- [ ] Stevia
- [ ] Shirataki/Miracle Noodles
- [ ] Other: _____
- [ ] Other: _____
- [ ] Other: _____

Calories: _____

DINNER Time :   WAS AN ITEM EATEN AS A SNACK? WHICH?   Time:

Protein:
- [ ] Chicken
- [ ] Beef
- [ ] Veal
- [ ] Shrimp
- [ ] Lobster
- [ ] White fish: _____
- [ ] Protein Shake
- [ ] Other: _____

Serving Size:
- [ ] 100 grams
- [ ] Other: _____

Calories: _____

Vegetable:
- [ ] Asparagus
- [ ] Beet Greens
- [ ] Cabbage
- [ ] Celery
- [ ] Chard
- [ ] Cucumber
- [ ] Fennel
- [ ] Lettuce
- [ ] Onions
- [ ] Radishes
- [ ] Spinach
- [ ] Tomatoes
- [ ] Other: _____
- [ ] Other: _____
- [ ] Other: _____

Calories: _____

Fruit:
- [ ] Strawberries
- [ ] ½ Grapefruit
- [ ] Apple
- [ ] Orange
- [ ] Other: _____

Starch:
- [ ] Grissini
- [ ] Melba
- [ ] Other: _____

Calories: _____

Other:
- [ ] TBS. Milk
- [ ] Juice of 1 Lemon
- [ ] Stevia
- [ ] Shirataki/Miracle Noodles
- [ ] Other: _____
- [ ] Other: _____
- [ ] Other: _____

Calories: _____

VLCD **25** (Date): _____

WEIGHT: _____

HCG DOSAGE: _____

HUNGER LEVEL: _____

BEDTIME/WAKE TIME: _____

HOURS SLEEP: _____

TOTAL CALORIES: _____

SUPPLEMENTS: _____

☐ Multivitamin ☐ B12 Shot ☐ Lipo Shot

INJECTION LOCATION   TIME: _____

☐ Belly ☐ Deltoid ☐ Thigh ☐ Other: _____

DROPS / PELLETS DOSE TIMING

1st Dose: _____   2nd Dose: _____

3rd Dose: _____   4th Dose: _____

PERSONAL NOTES

....

....

....

....

....

....

....

LIQUIDS:

4 LITERS	128 oz = 1 GALLON
3.5 LITERS	120 oz
3 LITERS	112 oz
2.5 LITERS	104 oz
2 LITERS	96 oz = 3 QUARTS
1.5 LITERS	88 oz
1 LITER	80 oz
.5 LITERS	72 oz
	64 oz = 2 QUARTS
	56 oz
	48 oz
	40 oz
	32 oz = 1 QUART
	24 oz
	16 oz
	8 oz = 1 CUP

BREAKFAST   Time :

☐ None ☐ Fruit: _____   ☐ Protein: _____   Calories: _____

Serving Size: _____   Serving Size: _____

LUNCH Time: _____

WAS AN ITEM EATEN AS A SNACK? WHICH?   Time: _____

Protein:
- ☐ Chicken breast
- ☐ Beef
- ☐ Veal
- ☐ Shrimp
- ☐ Lobster
- ☐ White fish: _____
- ☐ Protein Shake
- ☐ Other: _____

Serving Size:
- ☐ 100 grams/3.5 oz
- ☐ Other: _____

Vegetable:
- ☐ Asparagus
- ☐ Beet Greens
- ☐ Cabbage
- ☐ Celery
- ☐ Chard
- ☐ Cucumber
- ☐ Fennel
- ☐ Lettuce
- ☐ Onions
- ☐ Radishes
- ☐ Spinach
- ☐ Tomatoes
- ☐ Other: _____
- ☐ Other: _____
- ☐ Other: _____

Fruit:
- ☐ Strawberries
- ☐ ½ Grapefruit
- ☐ Apple
- ☐ Orange
- ☐ Other: _____

Starch:
- ☐ Grissini
- ☐ Melba
- ☐ Other: _____

Other:
- ☐ TBS. Milk
- ☐ Juice of 1 Lemon
- ☐ Stevia
- ☐ Shirataki/Miracle Noodles
- ☐ Other: _____
- ☐ Other: _____
- ☐ Other: _____

Calories: _____   Calories: _____   Calories: _____   Calories: _____

DINNER Time: _____

WAS AN ITEM EATEN AS A SNACK? WHICH?   Time: _____

Protein:
- ☐ Chicken
- ☐ Beef
- ☐ Veal
- ☐ Shrimp
- ☐ Lobster
- ☐ White fish: _____
- ☐ Protein Shake
- ☐ Other: _____

Serving Size:
- ☐ 100 grams
- ☐ Other: _____

Vegetable:
- ☐ Asparagus
- ☐ Beet Greens
- ☐ Cabbage
- ☐ Celery
- ☐ Chard
- ☐ Cucumber
- ☐ Fennel
- ☐ Lettuce
- ☐ Onions
- ☐ Radishes
- ☐ Spinach
- ☐ Tomatoes
- ☐ Other: _____
- ☐ Other: _____
- ☐ Other: _____

Fruit:
- ☐ Strawberries
- ☐ ½ Grapefruit
- ☐ Apple
- ☐ Orange
- ☐ Other: _____

Starch:
- ☐ Grissini
- ☐ Melba
- ☐ Other: _____

Other:
- ☐ TBS. Milk
- ☐ Juice of 1 Lemon
- ☐ Stevia
- ☐ Shirataki/Miracle Noodles
- ☐ Other: _____
- ☐ Other: _____
- ☐ Other: _____

Calories: _____   Calories: _____   Calories: _____   Calories: _____

HCGCHICA.COM – RAYZEL LAM   161

VLCD **26** (Date): _____

WEIGHT: _____

HCG DOSAGE: _____

HUNGER LEVEL: _____

BEDTIME/WAKE TIME: _____

HOURS SLEEP: _____

TOTAL CALORIES: _____

SUPPLEMENTS: _____

☐ Multivitamin ☐ B12 Shot ☐ Lipo Shot

INJECTION LOCATION   TIME: _____

☐ Belly ☐ Deltoid ☐ Thigh ☐ Other: _____

DROPS / PELLETS DOSE TIMING

1st Dose: _____   2nd Dose: _____

3rd Dose: _____   4th Dose: _____

PERSONAL NOTES

....

....

....

....

....

....

LIQUIDS:

4 LITERS	
3.5 LITERS	
3 LITERS	
2.5 LITERS	
2 LITERS	
1.5 LITERS	
1 LITER	
.5 LITERS	

128 oz = 1 GALLON
120 oz
112 oz
104 oz
96 oz = 3 QUARTS
88 oz
80 oz
72 oz
64 oz = 2 QUARTS
56 oz
48 oz
40 oz
32 oz = 1 QUART
24 oz
16 oz
8 oz = 1 CUP

BREAKFAST   Time :

☐ None ☐ Fruit: _____   ☐ Protein: _____   Calories: _____

Serving Size: _____   Serving Size: _____

LUNCH Time : .... WAS AN ITEM EATEN AS A SNACK? WHICH? .... Time:

Protein:
- ☐ Chicken breast
- ☐ Beef
- ☐ Veal
- ☐ Shrimp
- ☐ Lobster
- ☐ White fish: _____
- ☐ Protein Shake
- ☐ Other: _____

Serving Size:
- ☐ 100 grams/3.5 oz
- ☐ Other: _____

Calories: _____

Vegetable:
- ☐ Asparagus
- ☐ Beet Greens
- ☐ Cabbage
- ☐ Celery
- ☐ Chard
- ☐ Cucumber
- ☐ Fennel
- ☐ Lettuce
- ☐ Onions
- ☐ Radishes
- ☐ Spinach
- ☐ Tomatoes
- ☐ Other: _____
- ☐ Other: _____
- ☐ Other: _____

Calories: _____

Fruit:
- ☐ Strawberries
- ☐ ½ Grapefruit
- ☐ Apple
- ☐ Orange
- ☐ Other: _____

Starch:
- ☐ Grissini
- ☐ Melba
- ☐ Other: _____

Calories: _____

Other:
- ☐ TBS. Milk
- ☐ Juice of 1 Lemon
- ☐ Stevia
- ☐ Shirataki/Miracle Noodles
- ☐ Other: _____
- ☐ Other: _____
- ☐ Other: _____

Calories: _____

DINNER Time : .... WAS AN ITEM EATEN AS A SNACK? WHICH? .... Time:

Protein:
- ☐ Chicken
- ☐ Beef
- ☐ Veal
- ☐ Shrimp
- ☐ Lobster
- ☐ White fish: _____
- ☐ Protein Shake
- ☐ Other: _____

Serving Size:
- ☐ 100 grams
- ☐ Other: _____

Calories: _____

Vegetable:
- ☐ Asparagus
- ☐ Beet Greens
- ☐ Cabbage
- ☐ Celery
- ☐ Chard
- ☐ Cucumber
- ☐ Fennel
- ☐ Lettuce
- ☐ Onions
- ☐ Radishes
- ☐ Spinach
- ☐ Tomatoes
- ☐ Other: _____
- ☐ Other: _____
- ☐ Other: _____

Calories: _____

Fruit:
- ☐ Strawberries
- ☐ ½ Grapefruit
- ☐ Apple
- ☐ Orange
- ☐ Other: _____

Starch:
- ☐ Grissini
- ☐ Melba
- ☐ Other: _____

Calories: _____

Other:
- ☐ TBS. Milk
- ☐ Juice of 1 Lemon
- ☐ Stevia
- ☐ Shirataki/Miracle Noodles
- ☐ Other: _____
- ☐ Other: _____
- ☐ Other: _____

Calories: _____

VLCD **27** (Date): _____

WEIGHT: _____

HCG DOSAGE: _____

HUNGER LEVEL: _____

BEDTIME/WAKE TIME: _____

HOURS SLEEP: _____

TOTAL CALORIES: _____

SUPPLEMENTS: _____

☐ Multivitamin ☐ B12 Shot ☐ Lipo Shot

Often, it's not about becoming a new person, but becoming THE PERSON YOU were meant to be, and ALREADY ARE, but don't know how to be.
— Heath L. Buckmaster

INJECTION LOCATION   TIME: _____

☐ Belly ☐ Deltoid ☐ Thigh ☐ Other: _____

DROPS / PELLETS DOSE TIMING

1st Dose: _____   2nd Dose: _____

3rd Dose: _____   4th Dose: _____

PERSONAL NOTES

....
....
....
....
....
....
....

LIQUIDS:

4 LITERS		128 oz = 1 GALLON
3.5 LITERS		120 oz
3 LITERS		112 oz
2.5 LITERS		104 oz
2 LITERS		96 oz = 3 QUARTS
1.5 LITERS		88 oz
1 LITER		80 oz
.5 LITERS		72 oz
		64 oz = 2 QUARTS
		56 oz
		48 oz
		40 oz
		32 oz = 1 QUART
		24 oz
		16 oz
		8 oz = 1 CUP

BREAKFAST   Time : _____

☐ None ☐ Fruit: _____   ☐ Protein: _____   Calories: _____

Serving Size: _____   Serving Size: _____

LUNCH Time: _____

Time: _____

Protein:
- ☐ Chicken breast
- ☐ Beef
- ☐ Veal
- ☐ Shrimp
- ☐ Lobster
- ☐ White fish: _____
- ☐ Protein Shake
- ☐ Other: _____

Serving Size:
- ☐ 100 grams/3.5 oz
- ☐ Other: _____

Vegetable:
- ☐ Asparagus
- ☐ Beet Greens
- ☐ Cabbage
- ☐ Celery
- ☐ Chard
- ☐ Cucumber
- ☐ Fennel
- ☐ Lettuce
- ☐ Onions
- ☐ Radishes
- ☐ Spinach
- ☐ Tomatoes
- ☐ Other: _____
- ☐ Other: _____
- ☐ Other: _____

Fruit:
- ☐ Strawberries
- ☐ ½ Grapefruit
- ☐ Apple
- ☐ Orange
- ☐ Other: _____

Starch:
- ☐ Grissini
- ☐ Melba
- ☐ Other: _____

Other:
- ☐ TBS. Milk
- ☐ Juice of 1 Lemon
- ☐ Stevia
- ☐ Shirataki/Miracle Noodles
- ☐ Other: _____
- ☐ Other: _____
- ☐ Other: _____

Calories: _____   Calories: _____   Calories: _____   Calories: _____

DINNER Time: _____

Time: _____

Protein:
- ☐ Chicken
- ☐ Beef
- ☐ Veal
- ☐ Shrimp
- ☐ Lobster
- ☐ White fish: _____
- ☐ Protein Shake
- ☐ Other: _____

Serving Size:
- ☐ 100 grams
- ☐ Other: _____

Vegetable:
- ☐ Asparagus
- ☐ Beet Greens
- ☐ Cabbage
- ☐ Celery
- ☐ Chard
- ☐ Cucumber
- ☐ Fennel
- ☐ Lettuce
- ☐ Onions
- ☐ Radishes
- ☐ Spinach
- ☐ Tomatoes
- ☐ Other: _____
- ☐ Other: _____
- ☐ Other: _____

Fruit:
- ☐ Strawberries
- ☐ ½ Grapefruit
- ☐ Apple
- ☐ Orange
- ☐ Other: _____

Starch:
- ☐ Grissini
- ☐ Melba
- ☐ Other: _____

Other:
- ☐ TBS. Milk
- ☐ Juice of 1 Lemon
- ☐ Stevia
- ☐ Shirataki/Miracle Noodles
- ☐ Other: _____
- ☐ Other: _____
- ☐ Other: _____

Calories: _____   Calories: _____   Calories: _____   Calories: _____

VLCD **28** (Date): _____

WEIGHT: _____

HCG DOSAGE: _____

HUNGER LEVEL: _____

BEDTIME/WAKE TIME: _____

HOURS SLEEP: _____

TOTAL CALORIES: _____

SUPPLEMENTS: _____

☐ Multivitamin ☐ B12 Shot ☐ Lipo Shot

HCGCHICA TIP:

Break It Up

Some hCGers have jobs with long or odd hours. It can be helpful to spread your food out - even splitting your 100 gram protein into two 50 gram servings.

INJECTION LOCATION   TIME: _____

☐ Belly ☐ Deltoid ☐ Thigh ☐ Other: _____

DROPS / PELLETS DOSE TIMING

1st Dose: _____   2nd Dose: _____

3rd Dose: _____   4th Dose: _____

PERSONAL NOTES

· ·

....

....

....

....

....

....

....

LIQUIDS:

4 LITERS	
3.5 LITERS	
3 LITERS	
2.5 LITERS	
2 LITERS	
1.5 LITERS	
1 LITER	
.5 LITERS	

128 oz = 1 GALLON
120 oz
112 oz
104 oz
96 oz = 3 QUARTS
88 oz
80 oz
72 oz
64 oz = 2 QUARTS
56 oz
48 oz
40 oz
32 oz = 1 QUART
24 oz
16 oz
8 oz = 1 CUP

BREAKFAST   Time :

· ·

☐ None ☐ Fruit: _____   ☐ Protein: _____   Calories: _____

Serving Size: _____   Serving Size: _____

LUNCH Time: ____ WAS AN ITEM EATEN AS A SNACK? WHICH? Time: ____

Protein:
- ☐ Chicken breast
- ☐ Beef
- ☐ Veal
- ☐ Shrimp
- ☐ Lobster
- ☐ White fish: _____
- ☐ Protein Shake
- ☐ Other: _____

Serving Size:
- ☐ 100 grams/3.5 oz
- ☐ Other: _____

Calories: _____

Vegetable:
- ☐ Asparagus
- ☐ Beet Greens
- ☐ Cabbage
- ☐ Celery
- ☐ Chard
- ☐ Cucumber
- ☐ Fennel
- ☐ Lettuce
- ☐ Onions
- ☐ Radishes
- ☐ Spinach
- ☐ Tomatoes
- ☐ Other: _____
- ☐ Other: _____
- ☐ Other: _____

Calories: _____

Fruit:
- ☐ Strawberries
- ☐ ½ Grapefruit
- ☐ Apple
- ☐ Orange
- ☐ Other: _____

Starch:
- ☐ Grissini
- ☐ Melba
- ☐ Other: _____

Calories: _____

Other:
- ☐ TBS. Milk
- ☐ Juice of 1 Lemon
- ☐ Stevia
- ☐ Shirataki/Miracle Noodles
- ☐ Other: _____
- ☐ Other: _____
- ☐ Other: _____

Calories: _____

DINNER Time: ____ WAS AN ITEM EATEN AS A SNACK? WHICH? Time: ____

Protein:
- ☐ Chicken
- ☐ Beef
- ☐ Veal
- ☐ Shrimp
- ☐ Lobster
- ☐ White fish: _____
- ☐ Protein Shake
- ☐ Other: _____

Serving Size:
- ☐ 100 grams
- ☐ Other: _____

Calories: _____

Vegetable:
- ☐ Asparagus
- ☐ Beet Greens
- ☐ Cabbage
- ☐ Celery
- ☐ Chard
- ☐ Cucumber
- ☐ Fennel
- ☐ Lettuce
- ☐ Onions
- ☐ Radishes
- ☐ Spinach
- ☐ Tomatoes
- ☐ Other: _____
- ☐ Other: _____
- ☐ Other: _____

Calories: _____

Fruit:
- ☐ Strawberries
- ☐ ½ Grapefruit
- ☐ Apple
- ☐ Orange
- ☐ Other: _____

Starch:
- ☐ Grissini
- ☐ Melba
- ☐ Other: _____

Calories: _____

Other:
- ☐ TBS. Milk
- ☐ Juice of 1 Lemon
- ☐ Stevia
- ☐ Shirataki/Miracle Noodles
- ☐ Other: _____
- ☐ Other: _____
- ☐ Other: _____

Calories: _____

Reflections ON WEEK 4

REMEMBER, THIS IS NOT JUST ABOUT LOSING WEIGHT. IT'S ABOUT CHANGING YOUR WHOLE MINDSET ABOUT FOOD AND YOUR BODY.

YOU ARE BREAKING OLD PATTERNS RIGHT NOW. YOU ARE CREATING NEW PATTERNS. TRY NOT TO FOCUS YOUR PROGESS SOLELY ON WEIGHT LOSS.

SO WITH THAT IN MIND, HOW DID THIS WEEK GO?

What are you proud of? Why are you proud of it? What did you struggle with? What would you like to work on changing? What specific logical ways can you think of to make those adjustments? Or maybe you're just burned out at the moment - it's okay to just make it a rant.

....

....

....

....

....

....

....

....

....

....

....

....

....

....

....

....

Week 5

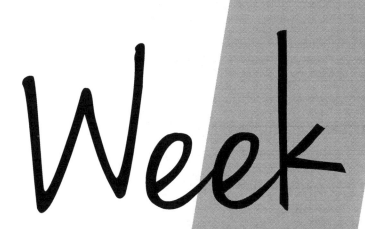

"WE HAVE TO ARTICULATE what we mean by change, define what we perceive as essential to our way of life. We have to refuse to accept blindly other's perceptions of progress."

– Patricia Locke, Lakota Indian

VLCD 29 (Date): _____

WEIGHT: _____

HCG DOSAGE: _____

HUNGER LEVEL: _____

BEDTIME/WAKE TIME: _____

HOURS SLEEP: _____

TOTAL CALORIES: _____

SUPPLEMENTS: _____

☐ Multivitamin   ☐ B12 Shot   ☐ Lipo Shot

INJECTION LOCATION   TIME: _____

☐ Belly   ☐ Deltoid   ☐ Thigh   ☐ Other: _____

DROPS / PELLETS DOSE TIMING

1st Dose: _____   2nd Dose: _____
3rd Dose: _____   4th Dose: _____

PERSONAL NOTES

....

....

....

....

....

....

....

LIQUIDS:

4 LITERS	128 oz = 1 GALLON
3.5 LITERS	120 oz
3 LITERS	112 oz
2.5 LITERS	104 oz
2 LITERS	96 oz = 3 QUARTS
1.5 LITERS	88 oz
1 LITER	80 oz
.5 LITERS	72 oz
	64 oz = 2 QUARTS
	56 oz
	48 oz
	40 oz
	32 oz = 1 QUART
	24 oz
	16 oz
	8 oz = 1 CUP

BREAKFAST   Time: _____

....

☐ None   ☐ Fruit: _____   ☐ Protein: _____   Calories: _____

Serving Size: _____   Serving Size: _____

LUNCH Time : Time:

Protein:
- [ ] Chicken breast
- [ ] Beef
- [ ] Veal
- [ ] Shrimp
- [ ] Lobster
- [ ] White fish: _____
- [ ] Protein Shake
- [ ] Other: _____

Serving Size:
- [ ] 100 grams/3.5 oz
- [ ] Other: _____

Calories: _____

Vegetable:
- [ ] Asparagus
- [ ] Beet Greens
- [ ] Cabbage
- [ ] Celery
- [ ] Chard
- [ ] Cucumber
- [ ] Fennel
- [ ] Lettuce
- [ ] Onions
- [ ] Radishes
- [ ] Spinach
- [ ] Tomatoes
- [ ] Other: _____
- [ ] Other: _____
- [ ] Other: _____

Calories: _____

Fruit:
- [ ] Strawberries
- [ ] ½ Grapefruit
- [ ] Apple
- [ ] Orange
- [ ] Other: _____

Starch:
- [ ] Grissini
- [ ] Melba
- [ ] Other: _____

Calories: _____

Other:
- [ ] TBS. Milk
- [ ] Juice of 1 Lemon
- [ ] Stevia
- [ ] Shirataki/Miracle Noodles
- [ ] Other: _____
- [ ] Other: _____
- [ ] Other: _____

Calories: _____

DINNER Time : Time:

Protein:
- [ ] Chicken
- [ ] Beef
- [ ] Veal
- [ ] Shrimp
- [ ] Lobster
- [ ] White fish: _____
- [ ] Protein Shake
- [ ] Other: _____

Serving Size:
- [ ] 100 grams
- [ ] Other: _____

Calories: _____

Vegetable:
- [ ] Asparagus
- [ ] Beet Greens
- [ ] Cabbage
- [ ] Celery
- [ ] Chard
- [ ] Cucumber
- [ ] Fennel
- [ ] Lettuce
- [ ] Onions
- [ ] Radishes
- [ ] Spinach
- [ ] Tomatoes
- [ ] Other: _____
- [ ] Other: _____
- [ ] Other: _____

Calories: _____

Fruit:
- [ ] Strawberries
- [ ] ½ Grapefruit
- [ ] Apple
- [ ] Orange
- [ ] Other: _____

Starch:
- [ ] Grissini
- [ ] Melba
- [ ] Other: _____

Calories: _____

Other:
- [ ] TBS. Milk
- [ ] Juice of 1 Lemon
- [ ] Stevia
- [ ] Shirataki/Miracle Noodles
- [ ] Other: _____
- [ ] Other: _____
- [ ] Other: _____

Calories: _____

VLCD 30 (Date): _____

WEIGHT: _____

HCG DOSAGE: _____

HUNGER LEVEL: _____

BEDTIME/WAKE TIME: _____

HOURS SLEEP: _____

TOTAL CALORIES: _____

SUPPLEMENTS: _____

☐ Multivitamin   ☐ B12 Shot   ☐ Lipo Shot

> Bad habits
> are like having a **SUMO WRESTLER**
> in the back of your canoe
> ROWING THE OPPOSITE DIRECTION.
> - J Loren Norris

INJECTION LOCATION   TIME: _____

☐ Belly   ☐ Deltoid   ☐ Thigh   ☐ Other: _____

DROPS / PELLETS DOSE TIMING

1st Dose: _____   2nd Dose: _____

3rd Dose: _____   4th Dose: _____

PERSONAL NOTES

....

....

....

....

....

....

....

....

LIQUIDS:

4 LITERS	128 oz = 1 GALLON
3.5 LITERS	120 oz
3 LITERS	112 oz
2.5 LITERS	104 oz
2 LITERS	96 oz = 3 QUARTS
1.5 LITERS	88 oz
1 LITER	80 oz
.5 LITERS	72 oz
	64 oz = 2 QUARTS
	56 oz
	48 oz
	40 oz
	32 oz = 1 QUART
	24 oz
	16 oz
	8 oz = 1 CUP

BREAKFAST   Time:

☐ None   ☐ Fruit: _____   ☐ Protein: _____   Calories: _____

Serving Size: _____   Serving Size: _____

LUNCH Time : _____

Protein:
- ☐ Chicken breast
- ☐ Beef
- ☐ Veal
- ☐ Shrimp
- ☐ Lobster
- ☐ White fish: _____
- ☐ Protein Shake
- ☐ Other: _____

Serving Size:
- ☐ 100 grams/3.5 oz
- ☐ Other: _____

Vegetable:
- ☐ Asparagus
- ☐ Beet Greens
- ☐ Cabbage
- ☐ Celery
- ☐ Chard
- ☐ Cucumber
- ☐ Fennel
- ☐ Lettuce
- ☐ Onions
- ☐ Radishes
- ☐ Spinach
- ☐ Tomatoes
- ☐ Other: _____
- ☐ Other: _____
- ☐ Other: _____

Fruit:
- ☐ Strawberries
- ☐ ½ Grapefruit
- ☐ Apple
- ☐ Orange
- ☐ Other: _____

Starch:
- ☐ Grissini
- ☐ Melba
- ☐ Other: _____

Other:
- ☐ TBS. Milk
- ☐ Juice of 1 Lemon
- ☐ Stevia
- ☐ Shirataki/Miracle Noodles
- ☐ Other: _____
- ☐ Other: _____
- ☐ Other: _____

Calories: _____   Calories: _____   Calories: _____   Calories: _____

DINNER Time : _____

Protein:
- ☐ Chicken
- ☐ Beef
- ☐ Veal
- ☐ Shrimp
- ☐ Lobster
- ☐ White fish: _____
- ☐ Protein Shake
- ☐ Other: _____

Serving Size:
- ☐ 100 grams
- ☐ Other: _____

Vegetable:
- ☐ Asparagus
- ☐ Beet Greens
- ☐ Cabbage
- ☐ Celery
- ☐ Chard
- ☐ Cucumber
- ☐ Fennel
- ☐ Lettuce
- ☐ Onions
- ☐ Radishes
- ☐ Spinach
- ☐ Tomatoes
- ☐ Other: _____
- ☐ Other: _____
- ☐ Other: _____

Fruit:
- ☐ Strawberries
- ☐ ½ Grapefruit
- ☐ Apple
- ☐ Orange
- ☐ Other: _____

Starch:
- ☐ Grissini
- ☐ Melba
- ☐ Other: _____

Other:
- ☐ TBS. Milk
- ☐ Juice of 1 Lemon
- ☐ Stevia
- ☐ Shirataki/Miracle Noodles
- ☐ Other: _____
- ☐ Other: _____
- ☐ Other: _____

Calories: _____   Calories: _____   Calories: _____   Calories: _____

VLCD 31 (Date): _____

WEIGHT: _____

HCG DOSAGE: _____

HUNGER LEVEL: _____

BEDTIME/WAKE TIME: _____

HOURS SLEEP: _____

TOTAL CALORIES: _____

SUPPLEMENTS: _____

☐ Multivitamin ☐ B12 Shot ☐ Lipo Shot

HCGCHICA TIP:

Start Looking Ahead

Towards the end of my rounds, I found it helpful and exciting to research recipes for Phase 3 on Pinterest that would replace my previous unhealthy stand-bys.

INJECTION LOCATION   TIME: _____

☐ Belly ☐ Deltoid ☐ Thigh ☐ Other: _____

DROPS / PELLETS DOSE TIMING

1st Dose: _____   2nd Dose: _____

3rd Dose: _____   4th Dose: _____

PERSONAL NOTES

....

....

....

....

....

....

....

LIQUIDS:

4 LITERS	128 oz = 1 GALLON
3.5 LITERS	120 oz
3 LITERS	112 oz
2.5 LITERS	104 oz
2 LITERS	96 oz = 3 QUARTS
1.5 LITERS	88 oz
1 LITER	80 oz
.5 LITERS	72 oz
	64 oz = 2 QUARTS
	56 oz
	48 oz
	40 oz
	32 oz = 1 QUART
	24 oz
	16 oz
	8 oz = 1 CUP

BREAKFAST   Time :

☐ None ☐ Fruit: _____   ☐ Protein: _____   *Calories:* _____

Serving Size: _____   *Serving Size:* _____

LUNCH Time: WAS AN ITEM EATEN AS A SNACK? WHICH?   Time:

Protein:
- [ ] Chicken breast
- [ ] Beef
- [ ] Veal
- [ ] Shrimp
- [ ] Lobster
- [ ] White fish: _____
- [ ] Protein Shake
- [ ] Other: _____

Serving Size:
- [ ] 100 grams/3.5 oz
- [ ] Other: _____

Vegetable:
- [ ] Asparagus
- [ ] Beet Greens
- [ ] Cabbage
- [ ] Celery
- [ ] Chard
- [ ] Cucumber
- [ ] Fennel
- [ ] Lettuce
- [ ] Onions
- [ ] Radishes
- [ ] Spinach
- [ ] Tomatoes
- [ ] Other: _____
- [ ] Other: _____
- [ ] Other: _____

Fruit:
- [ ] Strawberries
- [ ] ½ Grapefruit
- [ ] Apple
- [ ] Orange
- [ ] Other: _____

Starch:
- [ ] Grissini
- [ ] Melba
- [ ] Other: _____

Other:
- [ ] TBS. Milk
- [ ] Juice of 1 Lemon
- [ ] Stevia
- [ ] Shirataki/Miracle Noodles
- [ ] Other: _____
- [ ] Other: _____
- [ ] Other: _____

Calories: _____   Calories: _____   Calories: _____   Calories: _____

DINNER Time: WAS AN ITEM EATEN AS A SNACK? WHICH?   Time:

Protein:
- [ ] Chicken
- [ ] Beef
- [ ] Veal
- [ ] Shrimp
- [ ] Lobster
- [ ] White fish: _____
- [ ] Protein Shake
- [ ] Other: _____

Serving Size:
- [ ] 100 grams
- [ ] Other: _____

Vegetable:
- [ ] Asparagus
- [ ] Beet Greens
- [ ] Cabbage
- [ ] Celery
- [ ] Chard
- [ ] Cucumber
- [ ] Fennel
- [ ] Lettuce
- [ ] Onions
- [ ] Radishes
- [ ] Spinach
- [ ] Tomatoes
- [ ] Other: _____
- [ ] Other: _____
- [ ] Other: _____

Fruit:
- [ ] Strawberries
- [ ] ½ Grapefruit
- [ ] Apple
- [ ] Orange
- [ ] Other: _____

Starch:
- [ ] Grissini
- [ ] Melba
- [ ] Other: _____

Other:
- [ ] TBS. Milk
- [ ] Juice of 1 Lemon
- [ ] Stevia
- [ ] Shirataki/Miracle Noodles
- [ ] Other: _____
- [ ] Other: _____
- [ ] Other: _____

Calories: _____   Calories: _____   Calories: _____   Calories: _____

VLCD 32 (Date): _____

WEIGHT: _____

HCG DOSAGE: _____

HUNGER LEVEL: _____

BEDTIME/WAKE TIME: _____

HOURS SLEEP: _____

TOTAL CALORIES: _____

SUPPLEMENTS: _____

☐ Multivitamin   ☐ B12 Shot   ☐ Lipo Shot

> Sometimes,
> BEING TRUE to yourself
> means changing your mind.
> SELF CHANGES,
> and you follow.
> - Vera Nazarian

INJECTION LOCATION   TIME: _____

☐ Belly   ☐ Deltoid   ☐ Thigh   ☐ Other: _____

DROPS / PELLETS DOSE TIMING

1st Dose: _____   2nd Dose: _____
3rd Dose: _____   4th Dose: _____

PERSONAL NOTES

....
....
....
....
....
....
....

LIQUIDS:

4 LITERS	128 oz = 1 GALLON
3.5 LITERS	120 oz
3 LITERS	112 oz
2.5 LITERS	104 oz
2 LITERS	96 oz = 3 QUARTS
1.5 LITERS	88 oz
1 LITER	80 oz
.5 LITERS	72 oz
	64 oz = 2 QUARTS
	56 oz
	48 oz
	40 oz
	32 oz = 1 QUART
	24 oz
	16 oz
	8 oz = 1 CUP

BREAKFAST   Time:

☐ None   ☐ Fruit: _____   ☐ Protein: _____   Calories: _____
          Serving Size: _____   Serving Size: _____

LUNCH Time : _____   WAS AN ITEM EATEN AS A SNACK? WHICH?   Time: _____

Protein:
- [ ] Chicken breast
- [ ] Beef
- [ ] Veal
- [ ] Shrimp
- [ ] Lobster
- [ ] White fish: _____
- [ ] Protein Shake
- [ ] Other: _____

Serving Size:
- [ ] 100 grams/3.5 oz
- [ ] Other: _____

Vegetable:
- [ ] Asparagus
- [ ] Beet Greens
- [ ] Cabbage
- [ ] Celery
- [ ] Chard
- [ ] Cucumber
- [ ] Fennel
- [ ] Lettuce
- [ ] Onions
- [ ] Radishes
- [ ] Spinach
- [ ] Tomatoes
- [ ] Other: _____
- [ ] Other: _____
- [ ] Other: _____

Fruit:
- [ ] Strawberries
- [ ] ½ Grapefruit
- [ ] Apple
- [ ] Orange
- [ ] Other: _____

Starch:
- [ ] Grissini
- [ ] Melba
- [ ] Other: _____

Other:
- [ ] TBS. Milk
- [ ] Juice of 1 Lemon
- [ ] Stevia
- [ ] Shirataki/Miracle Noodles
- [ ] Other: _____
- [ ] Other: _____
- [ ] Other: _____

Calories: _____   Calories: _____   Calories: _____   Calories: _____

DINNER Time : _____   WAS AN ITEM EATEN AS A SNACK? WHICH?   Time: _____

Protein:
- [ ] Chicken
- [ ] Beef
- [ ] Veal
- [ ] Shrimp
- [ ] Lobster
- [ ] White fish: _____
- [ ] Protein Shake
- [ ] Other: _____

Serving Size:
- [ ] 100 grams
- [ ] Other: _____

Vegetable:
- [ ] Asparagus
- [ ] Beet Greens
- [ ] Cabbage
- [ ] Celery
- [ ] Chard
- [ ] Cucumber
- [ ] Fennel
- [ ] Lettuce
- [ ] Onions
- [ ] Radishes
- [ ] Spinach
- [ ] Tomatoes
- [ ] Other: _____
- [ ] Other: _____
- [ ] Other: _____

Fruit:
- [ ] Strawberries
- [ ] ½ Grapefruit
- [ ] Apple
- [ ] Orange
- [ ] Other: _____

Starch:
- [ ] Grissini
- [ ] Melba
- [ ] Other: _____

Other:
- [ ] TBS. Milk
- [ ] Juice of 1 Lemon
- [ ] Stevia
- [ ] Shirataki/Miracle Noodles
- [ ] Other: _____
- [ ] Other: _____
- [ ] Other: _____

Calories: _____   Calories: _____   Calories: _____   Calories: _____

VLCD 33 (Date): _____

WEIGHT: _____

HCG DOSAGE: _____

HUNGER LEVEL: _____

BEDTIME/WAKE TIME: _____

HOURS SLEEP: _____

TOTAL CALORIES: _____

SUPPLEMENTS: _____

☐ Multivitamin ☐ B12 Shot ☐ Lipo Shot

INJECTION LOCATION TIME: _____

☐ Belly ☐ Deltoid ☐ Thigh ☐ Other: _____

DROPS / PELLETS DOSE TIMING

1st Dose: _____   2nd Dose: _____

3rd Dose: _____   4th Dose: _____

PERSONAL NOTES

....

....

....

....

....

....

LIQUIDS:

4 LITERS	128 oz = 1 GALLON
3.5 LITERS	120 oz
3 LITERS	112 oz
2.5 LITERS	104 oz
2 LITERS	96 oz = 3 QUARTS
1.5 LITERS	88 oz
1 LITER	80 oz
.5 LITERS	72 oz
	64 oz = 2 QUARTS
	56 oz
	48 oz
	40 oz
	32 oz = 1 QUART
	24 oz
	16 oz
	8 oz = 1 CUP

BREAKFAST   Time :

☐ None ☐ Fruit: _____   ☐ Protein: _____   Calories: _____

Serving Size: _____   Serving Size: _____

LUNCH Time : _____

Protein:
- [ ] Chicken breast
- [ ] Beef
- [ ] Veal
- [ ] Shrimp
- [ ] Lobster
- [ ] White fish: _____
- [ ] Protein Shake
- [ ] Other: _____

Serving Size:
- [ ] 100 grams/3.5 oz
- [ ] Other: _____

Vegetable:
- [ ] Asparagus
- [ ] Beet Greens
- [ ] Cabbage
- [ ] Celery
- [ ] Chard
- [ ] Cucumber
- [ ] Fennel
- [ ] Lettuce
- [ ] Onions
- [ ] Radishes
- [ ] Spinach
- [ ] Tomatoes
- [ ] Other: _____
- [ ] Other: _____
- [ ] Other: _____

Fruit:
- [ ] Strawberries
- [ ] ½ Grapefruit
- [ ] Apple
- [ ] Orange
- [ ] Other: _____

Starch:
- [ ] Grissini
- [ ] Melba
- [ ] Other: _____

Other:
- [ ] TBS. Milk
- [ ] Juice of 1 Lemon
- [ ] Stevia
- [ ] Shirataki/Miracle Noodles
- [ ] Other: _____
- [ ] Other: _____
- [ ] Other: _____

Calories: _____   Calories: _____   Calories: _____   Calories: _____

DINNER Time : _____

Protein:
- [ ] Chicken
- [ ] Beef
- [ ] Veal
- [ ] Shrimp
- [ ] Lobster
- [ ] White fish: _____
- [ ] Protein Shake
- [ ] Other: _____

Serving Size:
- [ ] 100 grams
- [ ] Other: _____

Vegetable:
- [ ] Asparagus
- [ ] Beet Greens
- [ ] Cabbage
- [ ] Celery
- [ ] Chard
- [ ] Cucumber
- [ ] Fennel
- [ ] Lettuce
- [ ] Onions
- [ ] Radishes
- [ ] Spinach
- [ ] Tomatoes
- [ ] Other: _____
- [ ] Other: _____
- [ ] Other: _____

Fruit:
- [ ] Strawberries
- [ ] ½ Grapefruit
- [ ] Apple
- [ ] Orange
- [ ] Other: _____

Starch:
- [ ] Grissini
- [ ] Melba
- [ ] Other: _____

Other:
- [ ] TBS. Milk
- [ ] Juice of 1 Lemon
- [ ] Stevia
- [ ] Shirataki/Miracle Noodles
- [ ] Other: _____
- [ ] Other: _____
- [ ] Other: _____

Calories: _____   Calories: _____   Calories: _____   Calories: _____

VLCD 34 (Date): _____

WEIGHT: _____

HCG DOSAGE: _____

HUNGER LEVEL: _____

BEDTIME/WAKE TIME: _____

HOURS SLEEP: _____

TOTAL CALORIES: _____

SUPPLEMENTS: _____

☐ Multivitamin   ☐ B12 Shot   ☐ Lipo Shot

To PERSIST with a goal, you must TREASURE the dream more than the costs of sacrifice to ATTAIN it.
— Richelle E. Goodrich

INJECTION LOCATION   TIME: _____

☐ Belly   ☐ Deltoid   ☐ Thigh   ☐ Other: _____

DROPS / PELLETS DOSE TIMING

1st Dose: _____   2nd Dose: _____

3rd Dose: _____   4th Dose: _____

PERSONAL NOTES

....

....

....

....

....

....

....

LIQUIDS:

4 LITERS	128 oz = 1 GALLON
3.5 LITERS	120 oz
3 LITERS	112 oz
2.5 LITERS	104 oz
2 LITERS	96 oz = 3 QUARTS
1.5 LITERS	88 oz
1 LITER	80 oz
.5 LITERS	72 oz
	64 oz = 2 QUARTS
	56 oz
	48 oz
	40 oz
	32 oz = 1 QUART
	24 oz
	16 oz
	8 oz = 1 CUP

BREAKFAST   Time:

☐ None   ☐ Fruit: _____   ☐ Protein: _____   Calories: _____

Serving Size: _____   Serving Size: _____

LUNCH Time : _____ WAS AN ITEM EATEN AS A SNACK? WHICH? _____ Time: _____

Protein:
- ☐ Chicken breast
- ☐ Beef
- ☐ Veal
- ☐ Shrimp
- ☐ Lobster
- ☐ White fish: _____
- ☐ Protein Shake
- ☐ Other: _____

Serving Size:
- ☐ 100 grams/3.5 oz
- ☐ Other: _____

Calories: _____

Vegetable:
- ☐ Asparagus
- ☐ Beet Greens
- ☐ Cabbage
- ☐ Celery
- ☐ Chard
- ☐ Cucumber
- ☐ Fennel
- ☐ Lettuce
- ☐ Onions
- ☐ Radishes
- ☐ Spinach
- ☐ Tomatoes
- ☐ Other: _____
- ☐ Other: _____
- ☐ Other: _____

Calories: _____

Fruit:
- ☐ Strawberries
- ☐ ½ Grapefruit
- ☐ Apple
- ☐ Orange
- ☐ Other: _____

Starch:
- ☐ Grissini
- ☐ Melba
- ☐ Other: _____

Calories: _____

Other:
- ☐ TBS. Milk
- ☐ Juice of 1 Lemon
- ☐ Stevia
- ☐ Shirataki/Miracle Noodles
- ☐ Other: _____
- ☐ Other: _____
- ☐ Other: _____

Calories: _____

DINNER Time : _____ WAS AN ITEM EATEN AS A SNACK? WHICH? _____ Time: _____

Protein:
- ☐ Chicken
- ☐ Beef
- ☐ Veal
- ☐ Shrimp
- ☐ Lobster
- ☐ White fish: _____
- ☐ Protein Shake
- ☐ Other: _____

Serving Size:
- ☐ 100 grams
- ☐ Other: _____

Calories: _____

Vegetable:
- ☐ Asparagus
- ☐ Beet Greens
- ☐ Cabbage
- ☐ Celery
- ☐ Chard
- ☐ Cucumber
- ☐ Fennel
- ☐ Lettuce
- ☐ Onions
- ☐ Radishes
- ☐ Spinach
- ☐ Tomatoes
- ☐ Other: _____
- ☐ Other: _____
- ☐ Other: _____

Calories: _____

Fruit:
- ☐ Strawberries
- ☐ ½ Grapefruit
- ☐ Apple
- ☐ Orange
- ☐ Other: _____

Starch:
- ☐ Grissini
- ☐ Melba
- ☐ Other: _____

Calories: _____

Other:
- ☐ TBS. Milk
- ☐ Juice of 1 Lemon
- ☐ Stevia
- ☐ Shirataki/Miracle Noodles
- ☐ Other: _____
- ☐ Other: _____
- ☐ Other: _____

Calories: _____

VLCD **35** (Date): _____

WEIGHT: _____

HCG DOSAGE: _____

HUNGER LEVEL: _____

BEDTIME/WAKE TIME: _____

HOURS SLEEP: _____

TOTAL CALORIES: _____

SUPPLEMENTS: _____

☐ Multivitamin ☐ B12 Shot ☐ Lipo Shot

INJECTION LOCATION   TIME: _____

☐ Belly ☐ Deltoid ☐ Thigh ☐ Other: _____

DROPS / PELLETS DOSE TIMING

1st Dose: _____   2nd Dose: _____
3rd Dose: _____   4th Dose: _____

PERSONAL NOTES

....
....
....
....
....
....
....

LIQUIDS:

4 LITERS		128 oz = 1 GALLON
3.5 LITERS		120 oz
3 LITERS		112 oz
2.5 LITERS		104 oz
2 LITERS		96 oz = 3 QUARTS
1.5 LITERS		88 oz
1 LITER		80 oz
.5 LITERS		72 oz
		64 oz = 2 QUARTS
		56 oz
		48 oz
		40 oz
		32 oz = 1 QUART
		24 oz
		16 oz
		8 oz = 1 CUP

BREAKFAST   Time : _____

☐ None ☐ Fruit: _____ ☐ Protein: _____ Calories: _____

Serving Size: _____   Serving Size: _____

LUNCH Time :   WAS AN ITEM EATEN AS A SNACK? WHICH?   Time:

Protein:

- ☐ Chicken breast
- ☐ Beef
- ☐ Veal
- ☐ Shrimp
- ☐ Lobster
- ☐ White fish: _____
- ☐ Protein Shake
- ☐ Other: _____

Serving Size:
- ☐ 100 grams/3.5 oz
- ☐ Other: _____

Vegetable:

- ☐ Asparagus
- ☐ Beet Greens
- ☐ Cabbage
- ☐ Celery
- ☐ Chard
- ☐ Cucumber
- ☐ Fennel
- ☐ Lettuce
- ☐ Onions
- ☐ Radishes
- ☐ Spinach
- ☐ Tomatoes
- ☐ Other: _____
- ☐ Other: _____
- ☐ Other: _____

Fruit:

- ☐ Strawberries
- ☐ ½ Grapefruit
- ☐ Apple
- ☐ Orange
- ☐ Other: _____

Starch:

- ☐ Grissini
- ☐ Melba
- ☐ Other: _____

Other:

- ☐ TBS. Milk
- ☐ Juice of 1 Lemon
- ☐ Stevia
- ☐ Shirataki/Miracle Noodles
- ☐ Other: _____
- ☐ Other: _____
- ☐ Other: _____

Calories: _____   Calories: _____   Calories: _____   Calories: _____

DINNER Time :   WAS AN ITEM EATEN AS A SNACK? WHICH?   Time:

Protein:

- ☐ Chicken
- ☐ Beef
- ☐ Veal
- ☐ Shrimp
- ☐ Lobster
- ☐ White fish: _____
- ☐ Protein Shake
- ☐ Other: _____

Serving Size:
- ☐ 100 grams
- ☐ Other: _____

Vegetable:

- ☐ Asparagus
- ☐ Beet Greens
- ☐ Cabbage
- ☐ Celery
- ☐ Chard
- ☐ Cucumber
- ☐ Fennel
- ☐ Lettuce
- ☐ Onions
- ☐ Radishes
- ☐ Spinach
- ☐ Tomatoes
- ☐ Other: _____
- ☐ Other: _____
- ☐ Other: _____

Fruit:

- ☐ Strawberries
- ☐ ½ Grapefruit
- ☐ Apple
- ☐ Orange
- ☐ Other: _____

Starch:

- ☐ Grissini
- ☐ Melba
- ☐ Other: _____

Other:

- ☐ TBS. Milk
- ☐ Juice of 1 Lemon
- ☐ Stevia
- ☐ Shirataki/Miracle Noodles
- ☐ Other: _____
- ☐ Other: _____
- ☐ Other: _____

Calories: _____   Calories: _____   Calories: _____   Calories: _____

Reflections ON WEEK 5

REMEMBER, THIS IS NOT JUST ABOUT LOSING WEIGHT. IT'S ABOUT CHANGING YOUR WHOLE MINDSET ABOUT FOOD AND YOUR BODY,

YOU ARE BREAKING OLD PATTERNS RIGHT NOW. YOU ARE CREATING NEW PATTERNS. TRY NOT TO FOCUS YOUR PROGESS SOLELY ON WEIGHT LOSS.

SO WITH THAT IN MIND, HOW DID THIS WEEK GO?

What are you proud of? Why are you proud of it? What did you struggle with? What would you like to work on changing? What specific logical ways can you think of to make those adjustments? Or maybe you're just burned out at the moment - it's okay to just make it a rant.

....

....

....

....

....

....

....

....

....

....

....

....

....

....

....

Week 6

"I DID THEN WHAT I KNEW how to do. Now that I know better, I do better."

– Maya Angelou

VLCD **36** (Date): _____

WEIGHT: _____

HCG DOSAGE: _____

HUNGER LEVEL: _____

BEDTIME/WAKE TIME: _____

HOURS SLEEP: _____

TOTAL CALORIES: _____

SUPPLEMENTS: _____

☐ Multivitamin   ☐ B12 Shot   ☐ Lipo Shot

Many people succeed when OTHERS do not believe in them. But rarely does a person succeed when he does NOT BELIEVE IN HIMSELF.

- Herb True

INJECTION LOCATION   TIME: _____

☐ Belly   ☐ Deltoid   ☐ Thigh   ☐ Other: _____

DROPS / PELLETS DOSE TIMING

1st Dose: _____   2nd Dose: _____

3rd Dose: _____   4th Dose: _____

PERSONAL NOTES

....

....

....

....

....

....

LIQUIDS:

4 LITERS	128 oz = 1 GALLON
3.5 LITERS	120 oz
3 LITERS	112 oz
2.5 LITERS	104 oz
2 LITERS	96 oz = 3 QUARTS
1.5 LITERS	88 oz
1 LITER	80 oz
.5 LITERS	72 oz
	64 oz = 2 QUARTS
	56 oz
	48 oz
	40 oz
	32 oz = 1 QUART
	24 oz
	16 oz
	8 oz = 1 CUP

BREAKFAST   Time :

☐ None   ☐ Fruit: _____   ☐ Protein: _____   Calories: _____

Serving Size: _____   Serving Size: _____

LUNCH Time: _____

Protein:
- [ ] Chicken breast
- [ ] Beef
- [ ] Veal
- [ ] Shrimp
- [ ] Lobster
- [ ] White fish: _____
- [ ] Protein Shake
- [ ] Other: _____

Serving Size:
- [ ] 100 grams/3.5 oz
- [ ] Other: _____

Calories: _____

Vegetable:
- [ ] Asparagus
- [ ] Beet Greens
- [ ] Cabbage
- [ ] Celery
- [ ] Chard
- [ ] Cucumber
- [ ] Fennel
- [ ] Lettuce
- [ ] Onions
- [ ] Radishes
- [ ] Spinach
- [ ] Tomatoes
- [ ] Other: _____
- [ ] Other: _____
- [ ] Other: _____

Calories: _____

Fruit:
- [ ] Strawberries
- [ ] ½ Grapefruit
- [ ] Apple
- [ ] Orange
- [ ] Other: _____

Starch:
- [ ] Grissini
- [ ] Melba
- [ ] Other: _____

Calories: _____

Other:
- [ ] TBS. Milk
- [ ] Juice of 1 Lemon
- [ ] Stevia
- [ ] Shirataki/Miracle Noodles
- [ ] Other: _____
- [ ] Other: _____
- [ ] Other: _____

Calories: _____

DINNER Time: _____

Protein:
- [ ] Chicken
- [ ] Beef
- [ ] Veal
- [ ] Shrimp
- [ ] Lobster
- [ ] White fish: _____
- [ ] Protein Shake
- [ ] Other: _____

Serving Size:
- [ ] 100 grams
- [ ] Other: _____

Calories: _____

Vegetable:
- [ ] Asparagus
- [ ] Beet Greens
- [ ] Cabbage
- [ ] Celery
- [ ] Chard
- [ ] Cucumber
- [ ] Fennel
- [ ] Lettuce
- [ ] Onions
- [ ] Radishes
- [ ] Spinach
- [ ] Tomatoes
- [ ] Other: _____
- [ ] Other: _____
- [ ] Other: _____

Calories: _____

Fruit:
- [ ] Strawberries
- [ ] ½ Grapefruit
- [ ] Apple
- [ ] Orange
- [ ] Other: _____

Starch:
- [ ] Grissini
- [ ] Melba
- [ ] Other: _____

Calories: _____

Other:
- [ ] TBS. Milk
- [ ] Juice of 1 Lemon
- [ ] Stevia
- [ ] Shirataki/Miracle Noodles
- [ ] Other: _____
- [ ] Other: _____
- [ ] Other: _____

Calories: _____

VLCD 37 (Date): _____

WEIGHT: _____

HCG DOSAGE: _____

HUNGER LEVEL: _____

BEDTIME/WAKE TIME: _____

HOURS SLEEP: _____

TOTAL CALORIES: _____

SUPPLEMENTS: _____

☐ Multivitamin   ☐ B12 Shot   ☐ Lipo Shot

FELLOW HCGER TIP:

Shrimp WITH AN *Orange Twist*

Saute onion and garlic, add shrimp and cook just until turns pink. Eat with P2 orange slices.

INJECTION LOCATION   TIME: _____

☐ Belly   ☐ Deltoid   ☐ Thigh   ☐ Other: _____

DROPS / PELLETS DOSE TIMING

1st Dose: _____   2nd Dose: _____

3rd Dose: _____   4th Dose: _____

PERSONAL NOTES

....
....
....
....
....
....
....

LIQUIDS:

4 LITERS	128 oz = 1 GALLON
3.5 LITERS	120 oz
3 LITERS	112 oz
2.5 LITERS	104 oz
2 LITERS	96 oz = 3 QUARTS
1.5 LITERS	88 oz
1 LITER	80 oz
.5 LITERS	72 oz
	64 oz = 2 QUARTS
	56 oz
	48 oz
	40 oz
	32 oz = 1 QUART
	24 oz
	16 oz
	8 oz = 1 CUP

BREAKFAST   Time :

☐ None   ☐ Fruit: _____   ☐ Protein: _____   Calories: _____

Serving Size: _____   Serving Size: _____

LUNCH Time : ___

Protein:
- [ ] Chicken breast
- [ ] Beef
- [ ] Veal
- [ ] Shrimp
- [ ] Lobster
- [ ] White fish: _____
- [ ] Protein Shake
- [ ] Other: _____

Serving Size:
- [ ] 100 grams/3.5 oz
- [ ] Other: _____

Calories: _____

Vegetable:
- [ ] Asparagus
- [ ] Beet Greens
- [ ] Cabbage
- [ ] Celery
- [ ] Chard
- [ ] Cucumber
- [ ] Fennel
- [ ] Lettuce
- [ ] Onions
- [ ] Radishes
- [ ] Spinach
- [ ] Tomatoes
- [ ] Other: _____
- [ ] Other: _____
- [ ] Other: _____

Calories: _____

Fruit:
- [ ] Strawberries
- [ ] ½ Grapefruit
- [ ] Apple
- [ ] Orange
- [ ] Other: _____

Starch:
- [ ] Grissini
- [ ] Melba
- [ ] Other: _____

Calories: _____

Other:
- [ ] TBS. Milk
- [ ] Juice of 1 Lemon
- [ ] Stevia
- [ ] Shirataki/Miracle Noodles
- [ ] Other: _____
- [ ] Other: _____
- [ ] Other: _____

Calories: _____

DINNER Time : ___

Protein:
- [ ] Chicken
- [ ] Beef
- [ ] Veal
- [ ] Shrimp
- [ ] Lobster
- [ ] White fish: _____
- [ ] Protein Shake
- [ ] Other: _____

Serving Size:
- [ ] 100 grams
- [ ] Other: _____

Calories: _____

Vegetable:
- [ ] Asparagus
- [ ] Beet Greens
- [ ] Cabbage
- [ ] Celery
- [ ] Chard
- [ ] Cucumber
- [ ] Fennel
- [ ] Lettuce
- [ ] Onions
- [ ] Radishes
- [ ] Spinach
- [ ] Tomatoes
- [ ] Other: _____
- [ ] Other: _____
- [ ] Other: _____

Calories: _____

Fruit:
- [ ] Strawberries
- [ ] ½ Grapefruit
- [ ] Apple
- [ ] Orange
- [ ] Other: _____

Starch:
- [ ] Grissini
- [ ] Melba
- [ ] Other: _____

Calories: _____

Other:
- [ ] TBS. Milk
- [ ] Juice of 1 Lemon
- [ ] Stevia
- [ ] Shirataki/Miracle Noodles
- [ ] Other: _____
- [ ] Other: _____
- [ ] Other: _____

Calories: _____

VLCD **38** (Date): _____

WEIGHT: _____

HCG DOSAGE: _____

HUNGER LEVEL: _____

BEDTIME/WAKE TIME: _____

HOURS SLEEP: _____

TOTAL CALORIES: _____

SUPPLEMENTS: _____

☐ Multivitamin   ☐ B12 Shot   ☐ Lipo Shot

Failure should be our TEACHER, not our undertaker. Failure is DELAY, NOT DEFEAT. It is a temporary detour, NOT A DEAD END. Failure is something we can avoid only by saying nothing, doing nothing, and being nothing

- Denis Waitley

INJECTION LOCATION   TIME: _____

☐ Belly   ☐ Deltoid   ☐ Thigh   ☐ Other: _____

DROPS / PELLETS DOSE TIMING

1st Dose: _____   2nd Dose: _____

3rd Dose: _____   4th Dose: _____

PERSONAL NOTES

....

....

....

....

....

....

LIQUIDS:

4 LITERS	128 oz = 1 GALLON
3.5 LITERS	120 oz
3 LITERS	112 oz
2.5 LITERS	104 oz
2 LITERS	96 oz = 3 QUARTS
1.5 LITERS	88 oz
1 LITER	80 oz
.5 LITERS	72 oz
	64 oz = 2 QUARTS
	56 oz
	48 oz
	40 oz
	32 oz = 1 QUART
	24 oz
	16 oz
	8 oz = 1 CUP

BREAKFAST   Time :

☐ None   ☐ Fruit: _____   ☐ Protein: _____   Calories: _____

Serving Size: _____   Serving Size: _____

LUNCH Time :   WAS AN ITEM EATEN AS A SNACK? WHICH?   Time:

Protein:
- [ ] Chicken breast
- [ ] Beef
- [ ] Veal
- [ ] Shrimp
- [ ] Lobster
- [ ] White fish: _____
- [ ] Protein Shake
- [ ] Other: _____

Serving Size:
- [ ] 100 grams/3.5 oz
- [ ] Other: _____

Vegetable:
- [ ] Asparagus
- [ ] Beet Greens
- [ ] Cabbage
- [ ] Celery
- [ ] Chard
- [ ] Cucumber
- [ ] Fennel
- [ ] Lettuce
- [ ] Onions
- [ ] Radishes
- [ ] Spinach
- [ ] Tomatoes
- [ ] Other: _____
- [ ] Other: _____
- [ ] Other: _____

Fruit:
- [ ] Strawberries
- [ ] ½ Grapefruit
- [ ] Apple
- [ ] Orange
- [ ] Other: _____

Starch:
- [ ] Grissini
- [ ] Melba
- [ ] Other: _____

Other:
- [ ] TBS. Milk
- [ ] Juice of 1 Lemon
- [ ] Stevia
- [ ] Shirataki/Miracle Noodles
- [ ] Other: _____
- [ ] Other: _____
- [ ] Other: _____

Calories: _____   Calories: _____   Calories: _____   Calories: _____

DINNER Time :   WAS AN ITEM EATEN AS A SNACK? WHICH?   Time:

Protein:
- [ ] Chicken
- [ ] Beef
- [ ] Veal
- [ ] Shrimp
- [ ] Lobster
- [ ] White fish: _____
- [ ] Protein Shake
- [ ] Other: _____

Serving Size:
- [ ] 100 grams
- [ ] Other: _____

Vegetable:
- [ ] Asparagus
- [ ] Beet Greens
- [ ] Cabbage
- [ ] Celery
- [ ] Chard
- [ ] Cucumber
- [ ] Fennel
- [ ] Lettuce
- [ ] Onions
- [ ] Radishes
- [ ] Spinach
- [ ] Tomatoes
- [ ] Other: _____
- [ ] Other: _____
- [ ] Other: _____

Fruit:
- [ ] Strawberries
- [ ] ½ Grapefruit
- [ ] Apple
- [ ] Orange
- [ ] Other: _____

Starch:
- [ ] Grissini
- [ ] Melba
- [ ] Other: _____

Other:
- [ ] TBS. Milk
- [ ] Juice of 1 Lemon
- [ ] Stevia
- [ ] Shirataki/Miracle Noodles
- [ ] Other: _____
- [ ] Other: _____
- [ ] Other: _____

Calories: _____   Calories: _____   Calories: _____   Calories: _____

VLCD 39 (Date): _____

WEIGHT: _____

HCG DOSAGE: _____

HUNGER LEVEL: _____

BEDTIME/WAKE TIME: _____

HOURS SLEEP: _____

TOTAL CALORIES: _____

SUPPLEMENTS: _____

☐ Multivitamin   ☐ B12 Shot   ☐ Lipo Shot

FELLOW HCGER TIP:

Pre-frozen Lunch Bowls

Vicky says, "I make a huge batch of chicken and veggie soup at the beginning of every round and freeze in bowls. This way on the days I don't have time to fix a meal for work, I grab a bowl and it thaws by lunch time.

INJECTION LOCATION   TIME: _____

☐ Belly   ☐ Deltoid   ☐ Thigh   ☐Other: _____

DROPS / PELLETS DOSE TIMING

1st Dose: _____   2nd Dose: _____

3rd Dose: _____   4th Dose: _____

PERSONAL NOTES

· ·

....

....

....

....

....

....

....

LIQUIDS:

4 LITERS	128 oz = 1 GALLON
3.5 LITERS	120 oz
3 LITERS	112 oz
2.5 LITERS	104 oz
2 LITERS	96 oz = 3 QUARTS
1.5 LITERS	88 oz
1 LITER	80 oz
.5 LITERS	72 oz
	64 oz = 2 QUARTS
	56 oz
	48 oz
	40 oz
	32 oz = 1 QUART
	24 oz
	16 oz
	8 oz = 1 CUP

BREAKFAST   Time :

· ·

☐ None   ☐ Fruit: _____   ☐ Protein: _____   Calories: _____

Serving Size: _____   Serving Size: _____

LUNCH Time: WAS AN ITEM EATEN AS A SNACK? WHICH?   Time:

Protein:
- [ ] Chicken breast
- [ ] Beef
- [ ] Veal
- [ ] Shrimp
- [ ] Lobster
- [ ] White fish: _____
- [ ] Protein Shake
- [ ] Other: _____

Serving Size:
- [ ] 100 grams/3.5 oz
- [ ] Other: _____

Vegetable:
- [ ] Asparagus
- [ ] Beet Greens
- [ ] Cabbage
- [ ] Celery
- [ ] Chard
- [ ] Cucumber
- [ ] Fennel
- [ ] Lettuce
- [ ] Onions
- [ ] Radishes
- [ ] Spinach
- [ ] Tomatoes
- [ ] Other: _____
- [ ] Other: _____
- [ ] Other: _____

Fruit:
- [ ] Strawberries
- [ ] ½ Grapefruit
- [ ] Apple
- [ ] Orange
- [ ] Other: _____

Starch:
- [ ] Grissini
- [ ] Melba
- [ ] Other: _____

Other:
- [ ] TBS. Milk
- [ ] Juice of 1 Lemon
- [ ] Stevia
- [ ] Shirataki/Miracle Noodles
- [ ] Other: _____
- [ ] Other: _____
- [ ] Other: _____

Calories: _____   Calories: _____   Calories: _____   Calories: _____

DINNER Time: WAS AN ITEM EATEN AS A SNACK? WHICH?   Time:

Protein:
- [ ] Chicken
- [ ] Beef
- [ ] Veal
- [ ] Shrimp
- [ ] Lobster
- [ ] White fish: _____
- [ ] Protein Shake
- [ ] Other: _____

Serving Size:
- [ ] 100 grams
- [ ] Other: _____

Vegetable:
- [ ] Asparagus
- [ ] Beet Greens
- [ ] Cabbage
- [ ] Celery
- [ ] Chard
- [ ] Cucumber
- [ ] Fennel
- [ ] Lettuce
- [ ] Onions
- [ ] Radishes
- [ ] Spinach
- [ ] Tomatoes
- [ ] Other: _____
- [ ] Other: _____
- [ ] Other: _____

Fruit:
- [ ] Strawberries
- [ ] ½ Grapefruit
- [ ] Apple
- [ ] Orange
- [ ] Other: _____

Starch:
- [ ] Grissini
- [ ] Melba
- [ ] Other: _____

Other:
- [ ] TBS. Milk
- [ ] Juice of 1 Lemon
- [ ] Stevia
- [ ] Shirataki/Miracle Noodles
- [ ] Other: _____
- [ ] Other: _____
- [ ] Other: _____

Calories: _____   Calories: _____   Calories: _____   Calories: _____

VLCD **40** (Date): _____

WEIGHT: _____

HCG DOSAGE: _____

HUNGER LEVEL: _____

BEDTIME/WAKE TIME: _____

HOURS SLEEP: _____

TOTAL CALORIES: _____

SUPPLEMENTS: _____

☐ Multivitamin   ☐ B12 Shot   ☐ Lipo Shot

> Whenever you find yourself on the SIDE OF THE MAJORITY, it is time to PAUSE and reflect.
> - Mark Twain

INJECTION LOCATION   TIME: _____

☐ Belly   ☐ Deltoid   ☐ Thigh   ☐ Other: _____

DROPS / PELLETS DOSE TIMING

1st Dose: _____   2nd Dose: _____

3rd Dose: _____   4th Dose: _____

PERSONAL NOTES

....

....

....

....

....

....

....

LIQUIDS:

4 LITERS	128 oz = 1 GALLON
3.5 LITERS	120 oz
3 LITERS	112 oz
2.5 LITERS	104 oz
2 LITERS	96 oz = 3 QUARTS
1.5 LITERS	88 oz
1 LITER	80 oz
.5 LITERS	72 oz
	64 oz = 2 QUARTS
	56 oz
	48 oz
	40 oz
	32 oz = 1 QUART
	24 oz
	16 oz
	8 oz = 1 CUP

BREAKFAST   Time :

☐ None   ☐ Fruit: _____   ☐ Protein: _____   Calories: _____

Serving Size: _____   Serving Size: _____

LUNCH Time : 　　　WAS AN ITEM EATEN AS A SNACK? WHICH?　　　Time:

Protein:
- [ ] Chicken breast
- [ ] Beef
- [ ] Veal
- [ ] Shrimp
- [ ] Lobster
- [ ] White fish: _____
- [ ] Protein Shake
- [ ] Other: _____

Serving Size:
- [ ] 100 grams/3.5 oz
- [ ] Other: _____

Vegetable:
- [ ] Asparagus
- [ ] Beet Greens
- [ ] Cabbage
- [ ] Celery
- [ ] Chard
- [ ] Cucumber
- [ ] Fennel
- [ ] Lettuce
- [ ] Onions
- [ ] Radishes
- [ ] Spinach
- [ ] Tomatoes
- [ ] Other: _____
- [ ] Other: _____
- [ ] Other: _____

Fruit:
- [ ] Strawberries
- [ ] ½ Grapefruit
- [ ] Apple
- [ ] Orange
- [ ] Other: _____

Starch:
- [ ] Grissini
- [ ] Melba
- [ ] Other: _____

Other:
- [ ] TBS. Milk
- [ ] Juice of 1 Lemon
- [ ] Stevia
- [ ] Shirataki/Miracle Noodles
- [ ] Other: _____
- [ ] Other: _____
- [ ] Other: _____

Calories: _____ 　 Calories: _____ 　 Calories: _____ 　 Calories: _____

DINNER Time : 　　　WAS AN ITEM EATEN AS A SNACK? WHICH?　　　Time:

Protein:
- [ ] Chicken
- [ ] Beef
- [ ] Veal
- [ ] Shrimp
- [ ] Lobster
- [ ] White fish: _____
- [ ] Protein Shake
- [ ] Other: _____

Serving Size:
- [ ] 100 grams
- [ ] Other: _____

Vegetable:
- [ ] Asparagus
- [ ] Beet Greens
- [ ] Cabbage
- [ ] Celery
- [ ] Chard
- [ ] Cucumber
- [ ] Fennel
- [ ] Lettuce
- [ ] Onions
- [ ] Radishes
- [ ] Spinach
- [ ] Tomatoes
- [ ] Other: _____
- [ ] Other: _____
- [ ] Other: _____

Fruit:
- [ ] Strawberries
- [ ] ½ Grapefruit
- [ ] Apple
- [ ] Orange
- [ ] Other: _____

Starch:
- [ ] Grissini
- [ ] Melba
- [ ] Other: _____

Other:
- [ ] TBS. Milk
- [ ] Juice of 1 Lemon
- [ ] Stevia
- [ ] Shirataki/Miracle Noodles
- [ ] Other: _____
- [ ] Other: _____
- [ ] Other: _____

Calories: _____ 　 Calories: _____ 　 Calories: _____ 　 Calories: _____

FELLOW HCGER TIP:

"Apple Pie"

Slice an apple into tiny slices and put in a microwaveable dish. Add apple pie spice. Cover with a paper towel and microwave for 3 minutes.

VLCD **41** (Date): _____

WEIGHT: _____

HCG DOSAGE: _____

HUNGER LEVEL: _____

BEDTIME/WAKE TIME: _____

HOURS SLEEP: _____

TOTAL CALORIES: _____

SUPPLEMENTS: _____

☐ Multivitamin   ☐ B12 Shot   ☐ Lipo Shot

INJECTION LOCATION   TIME: _____

☐ Belly ☐ Deltoid ☐ Thigh ☐ Other: _____

DROPS / PELLETS DOSE TIMING

1st Dose: _____   2nd Dose: _____
3rd Dose: _____   4th Dose: _____

PERSONAL NOTES

....

....
....
....
....
....
....
....

LIQUIDS:

4 LITERS	128 oz = 1 GALLON
3.5 LITERS	120 oz
3 LITERS	112 oz
2.5 LITERS	104 oz
2 LITERS	96 oz = 3 QUARTS
1.5 LITERS	88 oz
1 LITER	80 oz
.5 LITERS	72 oz
	64 oz = 2 QUARTS
	56 oz
	48 oz
	40 oz
	32 oz = 1 QUART
	24 oz
	16 oz
	8 oz = 1 CUP

BREAKFAST   Time :

....

☐ None ☐ Fruit: _____   ☐ Protein: _____   *Calories:* _____
            Serving Size: _____   *Serving Size:* _____

LUNCH Time : _____   WAS AN ITEM EATEN AS A SNACK? WHICH?   Time: _____

Protein:
- [ ] Chicken breast
- [ ] Beef
- [ ] Veal
- [ ] Shrimp
- [ ] Lobster
- [ ] White fish: _____
- [ ] Protein Shake
- [ ] Other: _____

Serving Size:
- [ ] 100 grams/3.5 oz
- [ ] Other: _____

Calories: _____

Vegetable:
- [ ] Asparagus
- [ ] Beet Greens
- [ ] Cabbage
- [ ] Celery
- [ ] Chard
- [ ] Cucumber
- [ ] Fennel
- [ ] Lettuce
- [ ] Onions
- [ ] Radishes
- [ ] Spinach
- [ ] Tomatoes
- [ ] Other: _____
- [ ] Other: _____
- [ ] Other: _____

Calories: _____

Fruit:
- [ ] Strawberries
- [ ] ½ Grapefruit
- [ ] Apple
- [ ] Orange
- [ ] Other: _____

Starch:
- [ ] Grissini
- [ ] Melba
- [ ] Other: _____

Calories: _____

Other:
- [ ] TBS. Milk
- [ ] Juice of 1 Lemon
- [ ] Stevia
- [ ] Shirataki/Miracle Noodles
- [ ] Other: _____
- [ ] Other: _____
- [ ] Other: _____

Calories: _____

DINNER Time : _____   WAS AN ITEM EATEN AS A SNACK? WHICH?   Time: _____

Protein:
- [ ] Chicken
- [ ] Beef
- [ ] Veal
- [ ] Shrimp
- [ ] Lobster
- [ ] White fish: _____
- [ ] Protein Shake
- [ ] Other: _____

Serving Size:
- [ ] 100 grams
- [ ] Other: _____

Calories: _____

Vegetable:
- [ ] Asparagus
- [ ] Beet Greens
- [ ] Cabbage
- [ ] Celery
- [ ] Chard
- [ ] Cucumber
- [ ] Fennel
- [ ] Lettuce
- [ ] Onions
- [ ] Radishes
- [ ] Spinach
- [ ] Tomatoes
- [ ] Other: _____
- [ ] Other: _____
- [ ] Other: _____

Calories: _____

Fruit:
- [ ] Strawberries
- [ ] ½ Grapefruit
- [ ] Apple
- [ ] Orange
- [ ] Other: _____

Starch:
- [ ] Grissini
- [ ] Melba
- [ ] Other: _____

Calories: _____

Other:
- [ ] TBS. Milk
- [ ] Juice of 1 Lemon
- [ ] Stevia
- [ ] Shirataki/Miracle Noodles
- [ ] Other: _____
- [ ] Other: _____
- [ ] Other: _____

Calories: _____

VLCD 42 (Date): _____

WEIGHT: _____

HCG DOSAGE: _____

HUNGER LEVEL: _____

BEDTIME/WAKE TIME: _____

HOURS SLEEP: _____

TOTAL CALORIES: _____

SUPPLEMENTS: _____

☐ Multivitamin   ☐ B12 Shot   ☐ Lipo Shot

> *Change* is HARDEST at the beginning, *messiest* in the MIDDLE and BEST AT THE END.
> — Robin S. Sharma

INJECTION LOCATION   TIME: _____

☐ Belly   ☐ Deltoid   ☐ Thigh   ☐ Other: _____

DROPS / PELLETS DOSE TIMING

1st Dose: _____   2nd Dose: _____

3rd Dose: _____   4th Dose: _____

PERSONAL NOTES

....

....

....

....

....

....

....

LIQUIDS:

4 LITERS	128 oz = 1 GALLON
3.5 LITERS	120 oz
3 LITERS	112 oz
2.5 LITERS	104 oz
2 LITERS	96 oz = 3 QUARTS
1.5 LITERS	88 oz
1 LITER	80 oz
.5 LITERS	72 oz
	64 oz = 2 QUARTS
	56 oz
	48 oz
	40 oz
	32 oz = 1 QUART
	24 oz
	16 oz
	8 oz = 1 CUP

BREAKFAST   Time : _____

☐ None   ☐ Fruit: _____   ☐ Protein: _____   Calories: _____

Serving Size: _____   Serving Size: _____

LUNCH Time :

Time:

Protein:
- ☐ Chicken breast
- ☐ Beef
- ☐ Veal
- ☐ Shrimp
- ☐ Lobster
- ☐ White fish: _____
- ☐ Protein Shake
- ☐ Other: _____

Serving Size:
- ☐ 100 grams/3.5 oz
- ☐ Other: _____

Vegetable:
- ☐ Asparagus
- ☐ Beet Greens
- ☐ Cabbage
- ☐ Celery
- ☐ Chard
- ☐ Cucumber
- ☐ Fennel
- ☐ Lettuce
- ☐ Onions
- ☐ Radishes
- ☐ Spinach
- ☐ Tomatoes
- ☐ Other: _____
- ☐ Other: _____
- ☐ Other: _____

Fruit:
- ☐ Strawberries
- ☐ ½ Grapefruit
- ☐ Apple
- ☐ Orange
- ☐ Other: _____

Starch:
- ☐ Grissini
- ☐ Melba
- ☐ Other: _____

Other:
- ☐ TBS. Milk
- ☐ Juice of 1 Lemon
- ☐ Stevia
- ☐ Shirataki/Miracle Noodles
- ☐ Other: _____
- ☐ Other: _____
- ☐ Other: _____

Calories: _____   Calories: _____   Calories: _____   Calories: _____

DINNER Time :

Time:

Protein:
- ☐ Chicken
- ☐ Beef
- ☐ Veal
- ☐ Shrimp
- ☐ Lobster
- ☐ White fish: _____
- ☐ Protein Shake
- ☐ Other: _____

Serving Size:
- ☐ 100 grams
- ☐ Other: _____

Vegetable:
- ☐ Asparagus
- ☐ Beet Greens
- ☐ Cabbage
- ☐ Celery
- ☐ Chard
- ☐ Cucumber
- ☐ Fennel
- ☐ Lettuce
- ☐ Onions
- ☐ Radishes
- ☐ Spinach
- ☐ Tomatoes
- ☐ Other: _____
- ☐ Other: _____
- ☐ Other: _____

Fruit:
- ☐ Strawberries
- ☐ ½ Grapefruit
- ☐ Apple
- ☐ Orange
- ☐ Other: _____

Starch:
- ☐ Grissini
- ☐ Melba
- ☐ Other: _____

Other:
- ☐ TBS. Milk
- ☐ Juice of 1 Lemon
- ☐ Stevia
- ☐ Shirataki/Miracle Noodles
- ☐ Other: _____
- ☐ Other: _____
- ☐ Other: _____

Calories: _____   Calories: _____   Calories: _____   Calories: _____

Reflections ON WEEK 6

REMEMBER, THIS IS NOT JUST ABOUT LOSING WEIGHT. IT'S ABOUT CHANGING YOUR WHOLE MINDSET ABOUT FOOD AND YOUR BODY,

YOU ARE BREAKING OLD PATTERNS RIGHT NOW. YOU ARE CREATING NEW PATTERNS. TRY NOT TO FOCUS YOUR PROGESS SOLELY ON WEIGHT LOSS.

SO WITH THAT IN MIND, HOW DID THIS WEEK GO?

What are you proud of? Why are you proud of it? What did you struggle with? What would you like to work on changing? What specific logical ways can you think of to make those adjustments? Or maybe you're just burned out at the moment - it's okay to just make it a rant.

Week 7

"RESULTS FUEL BELIEF
which causes us
to take more action
and get more results."

-Todd Stocker

VLCD **43** (Date): _____

WEIGHT: _____

HCG DOSAGE: _____

HUNGER LEVEL: _____

BEDTIME/WAKE TIME: _____

HOURS SLEEP: _____

TOTAL CALORIES: _____

SUPPLEMENTS: _____

☐ Multivitamin ☐ B12 Shot ☐ Lipo Shot

FELLOW HCGER TIP:

Nifty Water Bead Tracker

Attach a water bead tracker to your water bottle to easily count the number of bottles you've drunk each day. Make your own by googling "water bead tracker tutorial."

INJECTION LOCATION   TIME: _____

☐ Belly ☐ Deltoid ☐ Thigh ☐ Other: _____

DROPS / PELLETS DOSE TIMING

1st Dose: _____   2nd Dose: _____

3rd Dose: _____   4th Dose: _____

PERSONAL NOTES

....

....

....

....

....

....

....

....

LIQUIDS:

4 LITERS	
3.5 LITERS	
3 LITERS	
2.5 LITERS	
2 LITERS	
1.5 LITERS	
1 LITER	
.5 LITERS	

128 oz = 1 GALLON	
120 oz	
112 oz	
104 oz	
96 oz = 3 QUARTS	
88 oz	
80 oz	
72 oz	
64 oz = 2 QUARTS	
56 oz	
48 oz	
40 oz	
32 oz = 1 QUART	
24 oz	
16 oz	
8 oz = 1 CUP	

BREAKFAST   Time : _____

☐ None ☐ Fruit: _____ ☐ Protein: _____ Calories: _____

Serving Size: _____   Serving Size: _____

LUNCH Time :

Protein:
- ☐ Chicken breast
- ☐ Beef
- ☐ Veal
- ☐ Shrimp
- ☐ Lobster
- ☐ White fish: _____
- ☐ Protein Shake
- ☐ Other: _____

Serving Size:
- ☐ 100 grams/3.5 oz
- ☐ Other: _____

Calories: _____

Vegetable:
- ☐ Asparagus
- ☐ Beet Greens
- ☐ Cabbage
- ☐ Celery
- ☐ Chard
- ☐ Cucumber
- ☐ Fennel
- ☐ Lettuce
- ☐ Onions
- ☐ Radishes
- ☐ Spinach
- ☐ Tomatoes
- ☐ Other: _____
- ☐ Other: _____
- ☐ Other: _____

Calories: _____

Fruit:
- ☐ Strawberries
- ☐ ½ Grapefruit
- ☐ Apple
- ☐ Orange
- ☐ Other: _____

Starch:
- ☐ Grissini
- ☐ Melba
- ☐ Other: _____

Calories: _____

Other:
- ☐ TBS. Milk
- ☐ Juice of 1 Lemon
- ☐ Stevia
- ☐ Shirataki/Miracle Noodles
- ☐ Other: _____
- ☐ Other: _____
- ☐ Other: _____

Calories: _____

DINNER Time :

Protein:
- ☐ Chicken
- ☐ Beef
- ☐ Veal
- ☐ Shrimp
- ☐ Lobster
- ☐ White fish: _____
- ☐ Protein Shake
- ☐ Other: _____

Serving Size:
- ☐ 100 grams
- ☐ Other: _____

Calories: _____

Vegetable:
- ☐ Asparagus
- ☐ Beet Greens
- ☐ Cabbage
- ☐ Celery
- ☐ Chard
- ☐ Cucumber
- ☐ Fennel
- ☐ Lettuce
- ☐ Onions
- ☐ Radishes
- ☐ Spinach
- ☐ Tomatoes
- ☐ Other: _____
- ☐ Other: _____
- ☐ Other: _____

Calories: _____

Fruit:
- ☐ Strawberries
- ☐ ½ Grapefruit
- ☐ Apple
- ☐ Orange
- ☐ Other: _____

Starch:
- ☐ Grissini
- ☐ Melba
- ☐ Other: _____

Calories: _____

Other:
- ☐ TBS. Milk
- ☐ Juice of 1 Lemon
- ☐ Stevia
- ☐ Shirataki/Miracle Noodles
- ☐ Other: _____
- ☐ Other: _____
- ☐ Other: _____

Calories: _____

VLCD **44** (Date): _____

> It is better
> to take MANY SMALL STEPS
> in the *right direction*
> than to make
> a great leap forward
> only to stumble backward.
> - Louis Sachar

WEIGHT: _____

HCG DOSAGE: _____

HUNGER LEVEL: _____

BEDTIME/WAKE TIME: _____

HOURS SLEEP: _____

TOTAL CALORIES: _____

SUPPLEMENTS: _____

☐ Multivitamin ☐ B12 Shot ☐ Lipo Shot

INJECTION LOCATION   TIME: _____

☐ Belly ☐ Deltoid ☐ Thigh ☐ Other: _____

DROPS / PELLETS DOSE TIMING

1st Dose: _____   2nd Dose: _____
3rd Dose: _____   4th Dose: _____

PERSONAL NOTES

....
....
....
....
....
....
....
....

LIQUIDS:

4 LITERS	
3.5 LITERS	
3 LITERS	
2.5 LITERS	
2 LITERS	
1.5 LITERS	
1 LITER	
.5 LITERS	

128 oz = 1 GALLON
120 oz
112 oz
104 oz
96 oz = 3 QUARTS
88 oz
80 oz
72 oz
64 oz = 2 QUARTS
56 oz
48 oz
40 oz
32 oz = 1 QUART
24 oz
16 oz
8 oz = 1 CUP

BREAKFAST   Time: _____

☐ None ☐ Fruit: _____   ☐ Protein: _____   Calories: _____
        Serving Size: _____   Serving Size: _____

LUNCH Time: _____

Protein:
- [ ] Chicken breast
- [ ] Beef
- [ ] Veal
- [ ] Shrimp
- [ ] Lobster
- [ ] White fish: _____
- [ ] Protein Shake
- [ ] Other: _____

Serving Size:
- [ ] 100 grams/3.5 oz
- [ ] Other: _____

Vegetable:
- [ ] Asparagus
- [ ] Beet Greens
- [ ] Cabbage
- [ ] Celery
- [ ] Chard
- [ ] Cucumber
- [ ] Fennel
- [ ] Lettuce
- [ ] Onions
- [ ] Radishes
- [ ] Spinach
- [ ] Tomatoes
- [ ] Other: _____
- [ ] Other: _____
- [ ] Other: _____

Fruit:
- [ ] Strawberries
- [ ] ½ Grapefruit
- [ ] Apple
- [ ] Orange
- [ ] Other: _____

Starch:
- [ ] Grissini
- [ ] Melba
- [ ] Other: _____

Other:
- [ ] TBS. Milk
- [ ] Juice of 1 Lemon
- [ ] Stevia
- [ ] Shirataki/Miracle Noodles
- [ ] Other: _____
- [ ] Other: _____
- [ ] Other: _____

Calories: _____   Calories: _____   Calories: _____   Calories: _____

DINNER Time: _____

Protein:
- [ ] Chicken
- [ ] Beef
- [ ] Veal
- [ ] Shrimp
- [ ] Lobster
- [ ] White fish: _____
- [ ] Protein Shake
- [ ] Other: _____

Serving Size:
- [ ] 100 grams
- [ ] Other: _____

Vegetable:
- [ ] Asparagus
- [ ] Beet Greens
- [ ] Cabbage
- [ ] Celery
- [ ] Chard
- [ ] Cucumber
- [ ] Fennel
- [ ] Lettuce
- [ ] Onions
- [ ] Radishes
- [ ] Spinach
- [ ] Tomatoes
- [ ] Other: _____
- [ ] Other: _____
- [ ] Other: _____

Fruit:
- [ ] Strawberries
- [ ] ½ Grapefruit
- [ ] Apple
- [ ] Orange
- [ ] Other: _____

Starch:
- [ ] Grissini
- [ ] Melba
- [ ] Other: _____

Other:
- [ ] TBS. Milk
- [ ] Juice of 1 Lemon
- [ ] Stevia
- [ ] Shirataki/Miracle Noodles
- [ ] Other: _____
- [ ] Other: _____
- [ ] Other: _____

Calories: _____   Calories: _____   Calories: _____   Calories: _____

VLCD **45** (Date): _____

WEIGHT: _____

HCG DOSAGE: _____

HUNGER LEVEL: _____

BEDTIME/WAKE TIME: _____

HOURS SLEEP: _____

TOTAL CALORIES: _____

SUPPLEMENTS: _____

☐ Multivitamin ☐ B12 Shot ☐ Lipo Shot

INJECTION LOCATION   TIME: _____

☐ Belly ☐ Deltoid ☐ Thigh ☐ Other: _____

DROPS / PELLETS DOSE TIMING

1st Dose: _____   2nd Dose: _____
3rd Dose: _____   4th Dose: _____

LIQUIDS:

4 LITERS	128 oz = 1 GALLON
3.5 LITERS	120 oz
3 LITERS	112 oz
2.5 LITERS	104 oz
2 LITERS	96 oz = 3 QUARTS
1.5 LITERS	88 oz
1 LITER	80 oz
.5 LITERS	72 oz
	64 oz = 2 QUARTS
	56 oz
	48 oz
	40 oz
	32 oz = 1 QUART
	24 oz
	16 oz
	8 oz = 1 CUP

PERSONAL NOTES

....

_____

_____

_____

_____

_____

_____

BREAKFAST   Time :

☐ None ☐ Fruit: _____   ☐ Protein: _____   Calories: _____

Serving Size: _____   Serving Size: _____

LUNCH Time: _____   WAS AN ITEM EATEN AS A SNACK? WHICH?   Time: _____

Protein:
- [ ] Chicken breast
- [ ] Beef
- [ ] Veal
- [ ] Shrimp
- [ ] Lobster
- [ ] White fish: _____
- [ ] Protein Shake
- [ ] Other: _____

Serving Size:
- [ ] 100 grams/3.5 oz
- [ ] Other: _____

Vegetable:
- [ ] Asparagus
- [ ] Beet Greens
- [ ] Cabbage
- [ ] Celery
- [ ] Chard
- [ ] Cucumber
- [ ] Fennel
- [ ] Lettuce
- [ ] Onions
- [ ] Radishes
- [ ] Spinach
- [ ] Tomatoes
- [ ] Other: _____
- [ ] Other: _____
- [ ] Other: _____

Fruit:
- [ ] Strawberries
- [ ] ½ Grapefruit
- [ ] Apple
- [ ] Orange
- [ ] Other: _____

Starch:
- [ ] Grissini
- [ ] Melba
- [ ] Other: _____

Other:
- [ ] TBS. Milk
- [ ] Juice of 1 Lemon
- [ ] Stevia
- [ ] Shirataki/Miracle Noodles
- [ ] Other: _____
- [ ] Other: _____
- [ ] Other: _____

Calories: _____   Calories: _____   Calories: _____   Calories: _____

DINNER Time: _____   WAS AN ITEM EATEN AS A SNACK? WHICH?   Time: _____

Protein:
- [ ] Chicken
- [ ] Beef
- [ ] Veal
- [ ] Shrimp
- [ ] Lobster
- [ ] White fish: _____
- [ ] Protein Shake
- [ ] Other: _____

Serving Size:
- [ ] 100 grams
- [ ] Other: _____

Vegetable:
- [ ] Asparagus
- [ ] Beet Greens
- [ ] Cabbage
- [ ] Celery
- [ ] Chard
- [ ] Cucumber
- [ ] Fennel
- [ ] Lettuce
- [ ] Onions
- [ ] Radishes
- [ ] Spinach
- [ ] Tomatoes
- [ ] Other: _____
- [ ] Other: _____
- [ ] Other: _____

Fruit:
- [ ] Strawberries
- [ ] ½ Grapefruit
- [ ] Apple
- [ ] Orange
- [ ] Other: _____

Starch:
- [ ] Grissini
- [ ] Melba
- [ ] Other: _____

Other:
- [ ] TBS. Milk
- [ ] Juice of 1 Lemon
- [ ] Stevia
- [ ] Shirataki/Miracle Noodles
- [ ] Other: _____
- [ ] Other: _____
- [ ] Other: _____

Calories: _____   Calories: _____   Calories: _____   Calories: _____

VLCD **46** (Date): _____

WEIGHT: _____

HCG DOSAGE: _____

HUNGER LEVEL: _____

BEDTIME/WAKE TIME: _____

HOURS SLEEP: _____

TOTAL CALORIES: _____

SUPPLEMENTS: _____

☐ Multivitamin ☐ B12 Shot ☐ Lipo Shot

Character

consists of what you **DO**

on the

THIRD AND FOURTH TRIES.

- James A. Michener

INJECTION LOCATION   TIME: _____

☐ Belly ☐ Deltoid ☐ Thigh ☐ Other: _____

DROPS / PELLETS DOSE TIMING

1st Dose: _____   2nd Dose: _____

3rd Dose: _____   4th Dose: _____

PERSONAL NOTES

....

....

....

....

....

....

....

LIQUIDS:

4 LITERS	128 oz = 1 GALLON
3.5 LITERS	120 oz
3 LITERS	112 oz
2.5 LITERS	104 oz
2 LITERS	96 oz = 3 QUARTS
1.5 LITERS	88 oz
1 LITER	80 oz
.5 LITERS	72 oz
	64 oz = 2 QUARTS
	56 oz
	48 oz
	40 oz
	32 oz = 1 QUART
	24 oz
	16 oz
	8 oz = 1 CUP

BREAKFAST   Time: ____

☐ None ☐ Fruit: _____   ☐ Protein: _____   *Calories:* _____

Serving Size: _____   Serving Size: _____

LUNCH Time: _____   WAS AN ITEM EATEN AS A SNACK? WHICH?   Time: _____

Protein:
- [ ] Chicken breast
- [ ] Beef
- [ ] Veal
- [ ] Shrimp
- [ ] Lobster
- [ ] White fish: _____
- [ ] Protein Shake
- [ ] Other: _____

Serving Size:
- [ ] 100 grams/3.5 oz
- [ ] Other: _____

Vegetable:
- [ ] Asparagus
- [ ] Beet Greens
- [ ] Cabbage
- [ ] Celery
- [ ] Chard
- [ ] Cucumber
- [ ] Fennel
- [ ] Lettuce
- [ ] Onions
- [ ] Radishes
- [ ] Spinach
- [ ] Tomatoes
- [ ] Other: _____
- [ ] Other: _____
- [ ] Other: _____

Fruit:
- [ ] Strawberries
- [ ] ½ Grapefruit
- [ ] Apple
- [ ] Orange
- [ ] Other: _____

Starch:
- [ ] Grissini
- [ ] Melba
- [ ] Other: _____

Other:
- [ ] TBS. Milk
- [ ] Juice of 1 Lemon
- [ ] Stevia
- [ ] Shirataki/Miracle Noodles
- [ ] Other: _____
- [ ] Other: _____
- [ ] Other: _____

Calories: _____   Calories: _____   Calories: _____   Calories: _____

DINNER Time: _____   WAS AN ITEM EATEN AS A SNACK? WHICH?   Time: _____

Protein:
- [ ] Chicken
- [ ] Beef
- [ ] Veal
- [ ] Shrimp
- [ ] Lobster
- [ ] White fish: _____
- [ ] Protein Shake
- [ ] Other: _____

Serving Size:
- [ ] 100 grams
- [ ] Other: _____

Vegetable:
- [ ] Asparagus
- [ ] Beet Greens
- [ ] Cabbage
- [ ] Celery
- [ ] Chard
- [ ] Cucumber
- [ ] Fennel
- [ ] Lettuce
- [ ] Onions
- [ ] Radishes
- [ ] Spinach
- [ ] Tomatoes
- [ ] Other: _____
- [ ] Other: _____
- [ ] Other: _____

Fruit:
- [ ] Strawberries
- [ ] ½ Grapefruit
- [ ] Apple
- [ ] Orange
- [ ] Other: _____

Starch:
- [ ] Grissini
- [ ] Melba
- [ ] Other: _____

Other:
- [ ] TBS. Milk
- [ ] Juice of 1 Lemon
- [ ] Stevia
- [ ] Shirataki/Miracle Noodles
- [ ] Other: _____
- [ ] Other: _____
- [ ] Other: _____

Calories: _____   Calories: _____   Calories: _____   Calories: _____

VLCD **47** (Date): _____

WEIGHT: _____

HCG DOSAGE: _____

HUNGER LEVEL: _____

BEDTIME/WAKE TIME: _____

HOURS SLEEP: _____

TOTAL CALORIES: _____

SUPPLEMENTS: _____

☐ Multivitamin   ☐ B12 Shot   ☐ Lipo Shot

INJECTION LOCATION   TIME: _____

☐ Belly   ☐ Deltoid   ☐ Thigh   ☐ Other: _____

DROPS / PELLETS DOSE TIMING

1st Dose: _____   2nd Dose: _____

3rd Dose: _____   4th Dose: _____

PERSONAL NOTES

· ·

....

....

....

....

....

....

LIQUIDS:

4 LITERS	128 oz = 1 GALLON
3.5 LITERS	120 oz
3 LITERS	112 oz
2.5 LITERS	104 oz
2 LITERS	96 oz = 3 QUARTS
1.5 LITERS	88 oz
1 LITER	80 oz
.5 LITERS	72 oz
	64 oz = 2 QUARTS
	56 oz
	48 oz
	40 oz
	32 oz = 1 QUART
	24 oz
	16 oz
	8 oz = 1 CUP

BREAKFAST   Time :

· ·

☐ None   ☐ Fruit: _____   ☐ Protein: _____   Calories: _____

Serving Size: _____   Serving Size: _____

LUNCH Time: ⟶ WAS AN ITEM EATEN AS A SNACK? WHICH? Time:

Protein:
- [ ] Chicken breast
- [ ] Beef
- [ ] Veal
- [ ] Shrimp
- [ ] Lobster
- [ ] White fish: _____
- [ ] Protein Shake
- [ ] Other: _____

Serving Size:
- [ ] 100 grams/3.5 oz
- [ ] Other: _____

Vegetable:
- [ ] Asparagus
- [ ] Beet Greens
- [ ] Cabbage
- [ ] Celery
- [ ] Chard
- [ ] Cucumber
- [ ] Fennel
- [ ] Lettuce
- [ ] Onions
- [ ] Radishes
- [ ] Spinach
- [ ] Tomatoes
- [ ] Other: _____
- [ ] Other: _____
- [ ] Other: _____

Fruit:
- [ ] Strawberries
- [ ] ½ Grapefruit
- [ ] Apple
- [ ] Orange
- [ ] Other: _____

Starch:
- [ ] Grissini
- [ ] Melba
- [ ] Other: _____

Other:
- [ ] TBS. Milk
- [ ] Juice of 1 Lemon
- [ ] Stevia
- [ ] Shirataki/Miracle Noodles
- [ ] Other: _____
- [ ] Other: _____
- [ ] Other: _____

Calories: _____ Calories: _____ Calories: _____ Calories: _____

DINNER Time: ⟶ WAS AN ITEM EATEN AS A SNACK? WHICH? Time:

Protein:
- [ ] Chicken
- [ ] Beef
- [ ] Veal
- [ ] Shrimp
- [ ] Lobster
- [ ] White fish: _____
- [ ] Protein Shake
- [ ] Other: _____

Serving Size:
- [ ] 100 grams
- [ ] Other: _____

Vegetable:
- [ ] Asparagus
- [ ] Beet Greens
- [ ] Cabbage
- [ ] Celery
- [ ] Chard
- [ ] Cucumber
- [ ] Fennel
- [ ] Lettuce
- [ ] Onions
- [ ] Radishes
- [ ] Spinach
- [ ] Tomatoes
- [ ] Other: _____
- [ ] Other: _____
- [ ] Other: _____

Fruit:
- [ ] Strawberries
- [ ] ½ Grapefruit
- [ ] Apple
- [ ] Orange
- [ ] Other: _____

Starch:
- [ ] Grissini
- [ ] Melba
- [ ] Other: _____

Other:
- [ ] TBS. Milk
- [ ] Juice of 1 Lemon
- [ ] Stevia
- [ ] Shirataki/Miracle Noodles
- [ ] Other: _____
- [ ] Other: _____
- [ ] Other: _____

Calories: _____ Calories: _____ Calories: _____ Calories: _____

VLCD **48** (Date): _____

> If you focus
> on results,
> you will never change.
> If you FOCUS ON CHANGE,
> you will get results.
> – Jack Dixon

WEIGHT: _____

HCG DOSAGE: _____

HUNGER LEVEL: _____

BEDTIME/WAKE TIME: _____

HOURS SLEEP: _____

TOTAL CALORIES: _____

SUPPLEMENTS: _____

☐ Multivitamin   ☐ B12 Shot   ☐ Lipo Shot

INJECTION LOCATION   TIME: _____

☐ Belly   ☐ Deltoid   ☐ Thigh   ☐ Other: _____

DROPS / PELLETS DOSE TIMING

1st Dose: _____   2nd Dose: _____
3rd Dose: _____   4th Dose: _____

PERSONAL NOTES

....
....
....
....
....
....
....

LIQUIDS:

4 LITERS		128 oz = 1 GALLON
3.5 LITERS		120 oz
3 LITERS		112 oz
2.5 LITERS		104 oz
2 LITERS		96 oz = 3 QUARTS
1.5 LITERS		88 oz
1 LITER		80 oz
.5 LITERS		72 oz
		64 oz = 2 QUARTS
		56 oz
		48 oz
		40 oz
		32 oz = 1 QUART
		24 oz
		16 oz
		8 oz = 1 CUP

BREAKFAST   Time :

☐ None   ☐ Fruit: _____   ☐ Protein: _____   Calories: _____
              Serving Size: _____   Serving Size: _____

LUNCH Time : _____

Time: _____

Protein:

- ☐ Chicken breast
- ☐ Beef
- ☐ Veal
- ☐ Shrimp
- ☐ Lobster
- ☐ White fish: _____
- ☐ Protein Shake
- ☐ Other: _____

Serving Size:
- ☐ 100 grams/3.5 oz
- ☐ Other: _____

Vegetable:

- ☐ Asparagus
- ☐ Beet Greens
- ☐ Cabbage
- ☐ Celery
- ☐ Chard
- ☐ Cucumber
- ☐ Fennel
- ☐ Lettuce
- ☐ Onions
- ☐ Radishes
- ☐ Spinach
- ☐ Tomatoes
- ☐ Other: _____
- ☐ Other: _____
- ☐ Other: _____

Fruit:

- ☐ Strawberries
- ☐ ½ Grapefruit
- ☐ Apple
- ☐ Orange
- ☐ Other: _____

Starch:

- ☐ Grissini
- ☐ Melba
- ☐ Other: _____

Other:

- ☐ TBS. Milk
- ☐ Juice of 1 Lemon
- ☐ Stevia
- ☐ Shirataki/Miracle Noodles
- ☐ Other: _____
- ☐ Other: _____
- ☐ Other: _____

Calories: _____   Calories: _____   Calories: _____   Calories: _____

DINNER Time : _____

Time: _____

Protein:

- ☐ Chicken
- ☐ Beef
- ☐ Veal
- ☐ Shrimp
- ☐ Lobster
- ☐ White fish: _____
- ☐ Protein Shake
- ☐ Other: _____

Serving Size:
- ☐ 100 grams
- ☐ Other: _____

Vegetable:

- ☐ Asparagus
- ☐ Beet Greens
- ☐ Cabbage
- ☐ Celery
- ☐ Chard
- ☐ Cucumber
- ☐ Fennel
- ☐ Lettuce
- ☐ Onions
- ☐ Radishes
- ☐ Spinach
- ☐ Tomatoes
- ☐ Other: _____
- ☐ Other: _____
- ☐ Other: _____

Fruit:

- ☐ Strawberries
- ☐ ½ Grapefruit
- ☐ Apple
- ☐ Orange
- ☐ Other: _____

Starch:

- ☐ Grissini
- ☐ Melba
- ☐ Other: _____

Other:

- ☐ TBS. Milk
- ☐ Juice of 1 Lemon
- ☐ Stevia
- ☐ Shirataki/Miracle Noodles
- ☐ Other: _____
- ☐ Other: _____
- ☐ Other: _____

Calories: _____   Calories: _____   Calories: _____   Calories: _____

VLCD **49** (Date): _____

WEIGHT: _____

HCG DOSAGE: _____

HUNGER LEVEL: _____

BEDTIME/WAKE TIME: _____

HOURS SLEEP: _____

TOTAL CALORIES: _____

SUPPLEMENTS: _____

☐ Multivitamin   ☐ B12 Shot   ☐ Lipo Shot

INJECTION LOCATION   TIME: _____

☐ Belly   ☐ Deltoid   ☐ Thigh   ☐ Other: _____

DROPS / PELLETS DOSE TIMING

1st Dose: _____   2nd Dose: _____

3rd Dose: _____   4th Dose: _____

PERSONAL NOTES

....

....

....

....

....

....

....

LIQUIDS:

4 LITERS
3.5 LITERS
3 LITERS
2.5 LITERS
2 LITERS
1.5 LITERS
1 LITER
.5 LITERS

128 oz = 1 GALLON
120 oz
112 oz
104 oz
96 oz = 3 QUARTS
88 oz
80 oz
72 oz
64 oz = 2 QUARTS
56 oz
48 oz
40 oz
32 oz = 1 QUART
24 oz
16 oz
8 oz = 1 CUP

BREAKFAST   Time :

☐ None   ☐ Fruit: _____   ☐ Protein: _____   Calories: _____

Serving Size: _____   Serving Size: _____

LUNCH Time :   Time:

Protein:
- ☐ Chicken breast
- ☐ Beef
- ☐ Veal
- ☐ Shrimp
- ☐ Lobster
- ☐ White fish: _____
- ☐ Protein Shake
- ☐ Other: _____

Serving Size:
- ☐ 100 grams/3.5 oz
- ☐ Other: _____

Vegetable:
- ☐ Asparagus
- ☐ Beet Greens
- ☐ Cabbage
- ☐ Celery
- ☐ Chard
- ☐ Cucumber
- ☐ Fennel
- ☐ Lettuce
- ☐ Onions
- ☐ Radishes
- ☐ Spinach
- ☐ Tomatoes
- ☐ Other: _____
- ☐ Other: _____
- ☐ Other: _____

Fruit:
- ☐ Strawberries
- ☐ ½ Grapefruit
- ☐ Apple
- ☐ Orange
- ☐ Other: _____

Starch:
- ☐ Grissini
- ☐ Melba
- ☐ Other: _____

Other:
- ☐ TBS. Milk
- ☐ Juice of 1 Lemon
- ☐ Stevia
- ☐ Shirataki/Miracle Noodles
- ☐ Other: _____
- ☐ Other: _____
- ☐ Other: _____

Calories: _____   Calories: _____   Calories: _____   Calories: _____

DINNER Time :   Time:

Protein:
- ☐ Chicken
- ☐ Beef
- ☐ Veal
- ☐ Shrimp
- ☐ Lobster
- ☐ White fish: _____
- ☐ Protein Shake
- ☐ Other: _____

Serving Size:
- ☐ 100 grams
- ☐ Other: _____

Vegetable:
- ☐ Asparagus
- ☐ Beet Greens
- ☐ Cabbage
- ☐ Celery
- ☐ Chard
- ☐ Cucumber
- ☐ Fennel
- ☐ Lettuce
- ☐ Onions
- ☐ Radishes
- ☐ Spinach
- ☐ Tomatoes
- ☐ Other: _____
- ☐ Other: _____
- ☐ Other: _____

Fruit:
- ☐ Strawberries
- ☐ ½ Grapefruit
- ☐ Apple
- ☐ Orange
- ☐ Other: _____

Starch:
- ☐ Grissini
- ☐ Melba
- ☐ Other: _____

Other:
- ☐ TBS. Milk
- ☐ Juice of 1 Lemon
- ☐ Stevia
- ☐ Shirataki/Miracle Noodles
- ☐ Other: _____
- ☐ Other: _____
- ☐ Other: _____

Calories: _____   Calories: _____   Calories: _____   Calories: _____

Reflections ON WEEK 7

REMEMBER, THIS IS NOT JUST ABOUT LOSING WEIGHT. IT'S ABOUT CHANGING YOUR WHOLE MINDSET ABOUT FOOD AND YOUR BODY,

YOU ARE BREAKING OLD PATTERNS RIGHT NOW. YOU ARE CREATING NEW PATTERNS. TRY NOT TO FOCUS YOUR PROGESS SOLELY ON WEIGHT LOSS.

SO WITH THAT IN MIND, HOW DID THIS WEEK GO?

What are you proud of? Why are you proud of it? What did you struggle with? What would you like to work on changing? What specific logical ways can you think of to make those adjustments? Or maybe you're just burned out at the moment - it's okay to just make it a rant.

Week 8

"I LEARNED THAT we can do anything, but we can't do everything...at least not at the same time. So think of your priorities not in terms of what activities you do, but when you do them. Timing is everything."

— Dan Millman

> The pessimist complains about the wind; the optimist expects it to change; the realist ADJUSTS THE SAILS.
>
> *- Ralph Waldo Emerson*

VLCD 50 (Date): _____

WEIGHT: _____

HCG DOSAGE: _____

HUNGER LEVEL: _____

BEDTIME/WAKE TIME: _____

HOURS SLEEP: _____

TOTAL CALORIES: _____

SUPPLEMENTS: _____

☐ Multivitamin ☐ B12 Shot ☐ Lipo Shot

INJECTION LOCATION   TIME: _____

☐ Belly ☐ Deltoid ☐ Thigh ☐ Other: _____

DROPS / PELLETS DOSE TIMING

1st Dose: _____ 2nd Dose: _____

3rd Dose: _____ 4th Dose: _____

PERSONAL NOTES

....

....

....

....

....

....

....

LIQUIDS:

4 LITERS	128 oz = 1 GALLON
3.5 LITERS	120 oz
3 LITERS	112 oz
2.5 LITERS	104 oz
2 LITERS	96 oz = 3 QUARTS
1.5 LITERS	88 oz
1 LITER	80 oz
.5 LITERS	72 oz
	64 oz = 2 QUARTS
	56 oz
	48 oz
	40 oz
	32 oz = 1 QUART
	24 oz
	16 oz
	8 oz = 1 CUP

BREAKFAST   *Time :*

☐ None ☐ Fruit: _____ ☐ Protein: _____   *Calories:* _____

Serving Size: _____   Serving Size: _____

LUNCH Time :

Protein:
- [ ] Chicken breast
- [ ] Beef
- [ ] Veal
- [ ] Shrimp
- [ ] Lobster
- [ ] White fish: _____
- [ ] Protein Shake
- [ ] Other: _____

Serving Size:
- [ ] 100 grams/3.5 oz
- [ ] Other: _____

Calories: _____

Vegetable:
- [ ] Asparagus
- [ ] Beet Greens
- [ ] Cabbage
- [ ] Celery
- [ ] Chard
- [ ] Cucumber
- [ ] Fennel
- [ ] Lettuce
- [ ] Onions
- [ ] Radishes
- [ ] Spinach
- [ ] Tomatoes
- [ ] Other: _____
- [ ] Other: _____
- [ ] Other: _____

Calories: _____

Fruit:
- [ ] Strawberries
- [ ] ½ Grapefruit
- [ ] Apple
- [ ] Orange
- [ ] Other: _____

Starch:
- [ ] Grissini
- [ ] Melba
- [ ] Other: _____

Calories: _____

Other:
- [ ] TBS. Milk
- [ ] Juice of 1 Lemon
- [ ] Stevia
- [ ] Shirataki/Miracle Noodles
- [ ] Other: _____
- [ ] Other: _____
- [ ] Other: _____

Calories: _____

DINNER Time :

Protein:
- [ ] Chicken
- [ ] Beef
- [ ] Veal
- [ ] Shrimp
- [ ] Lobster
- [ ] White fish: _____
- [ ] Protein Shake
- [ ] Other: _____

Serving Size:
- [ ] 100 grams
- [ ] Other: _____

Calories: _____

Vegetable:
- [ ] Asparagus
- [ ] Beet Greens
- [ ] Cabbage
- [ ] Celery
- [ ] Chard
- [ ] Cucumber
- [ ] Fennel
- [ ] Lettuce
- [ ] Onions
- [ ] Radishes
- [ ] Spinach
- [ ] Tomatoes
- [ ] Other: _____
- [ ] Other: _____
- [ ] Other: _____

Calories: _____

Fruit:
- [ ] Strawberries
- [ ] ½ Grapefruit
- [ ] Apple
- [ ] Orange
- [ ] Other: _____

Starch:
- [ ] Grissini
- [ ] Melba
- [ ] Other: _____

Calories: _____

Other:
- [ ] TBS. Milk
- [ ] Juice of 1 Lemon
- [ ] Stevia
- [ ] Shirataki/Miracle Noodles
- [ ] Other: _____
- [ ] Other: _____
- [ ] Other: _____

Calories: _____

FELLOW HCGER TIP:

Crab Cakes Recipe

100 grams lump crab meat, 1 crumbled grissini or melba, 2 tbs. chopped dill, salt, pepper, tbs. seafood seasoning, 1 tbs. mustard.
Make into patties and heat in pan until browned on both sides.

WEIGHT: _____

HCG DOSAGE: _____

HUNGER LEVEL: _____

BEDTIME/WAKE TIME: _____

HOURS SLEEP: _____

TOTAL CALORIES: _____

SUPPLEMENTS: _____

☐ Multivitamin ☐ B12 Shot ☐ Lipo Shot

INJECTION LOCATION TIME: _____

☐ Belly ☐ Deltoid ☐ Thigh ☐ Other: _____

DROPS / PELLETS DOSE TIMING

1st Dose: _____   2nd Dose: _____
3rd Dose: _____   4th Dose: _____

PERSONAL NOTES

....
....
....
....
....
....
....

LIQUIDS:

4 LITERS	128 oz = 1 GALLON
3.5 LITERS	120 oz
3 LITERS	112 oz
2.5 LITERS	104 oz
2 LITERS	96 oz = 3 QUARTS
1.5 LITERS	88 oz
1 LITER	80 oz
.5 LITERS	72 oz
	64 oz = 2 QUARTS
	56 oz
	48 oz
	40 oz
	32 oz = 1 QUART
	24 oz
	16 oz
	8 oz = 1 CUP

BREAKFAST *Time* :

☐ None ☐ Fruit: _____ ☐ Protein: _____ *Calories*: _____
            Serving Size: _____ Serving Size: _____

LUNCH Time :

Time:

Protein:
- [ ] Chicken breast
- [ ] Beef
- [ ] Veal
- [ ] Shrimp
- [ ] Lobster
- [ ] White fish: _____
- [ ] Protein Shake
- [ ] Other: _____

Serving Size:
- [ ] 100 grams/3.5 oz
- [ ] Other: _____

Vegetable:
- [ ] Asparagus
- [ ] Beet Greens
- [ ] Cabbage
- [ ] Celery
- [ ] Chard
- [ ] Cucumber
- [ ] Fennel
- [ ] Lettuce
- [ ] Onions
- [ ] Radishes
- [ ] Spinach
- [ ] Tomatoes
- [ ] Other: _____
- [ ] Other: _____
- [ ] Other: _____

Fruit:
- [ ] Strawberries
- [ ] ½ Grapefruit
- [ ] Apple
- [ ] Orange
- [ ] Other: _____

Starch:
- [ ] Grissini
- [ ] Melba
- [ ] Other: _____

Other:
- [ ] TBS. Milk
- [ ] Juice of 1 Lemon
- [ ] Stevia
- [ ] Shirataki/Miracle Noodles
- [ ] Other: _____
- [ ] Other: _____
- [ ] Other: _____

Calories: _____   Calories: _____   Calories: _____   Calories: _____

DINNER Time :

Time:

Protein:
- [ ] Chicken
- [ ] Beef
- [ ] Veal
- [ ] Shrimp
- [ ] Lobster
- [ ] White fish: _____
- [ ] Protein Shake
- [ ] Other: _____

Serving Size:
- [ ] 100 grams
- [ ] Other: _____

Vegetable:
- [ ] Asparagus
- [ ] Beet Greens
- [ ] Cabbage
- [ ] Celery
- [ ] Chard
- [ ] Cucumber
- [ ] Fennel
- [ ] Lettuce
- [ ] Onions
- [ ] Radishes
- [ ] Spinach
- [ ] Tomatoes
- [ ] Other: _____
- [ ] Other: _____
- [ ] Other: _____

Fruit:
- [ ] Strawberries
- [ ] ½ Grapefruit
- [ ] Apple
- [ ] Orange
- [ ] Other: _____

Starch:
- [ ] Grissini
- [ ] Melba
- [ ] Other: _____

Other:
- [ ] TBS. Milk
- [ ] Juice of 1 Lemon
- [ ] Stevia
- [ ] Shirataki/Miracle Noodles
- [ ] Other: _____
- [ ] Other: _____
- [ ] Other: _____

Calories: _____   Calories: _____   Calories: _____   Calories: _____

VLCD **52** (Date): _____

WEIGHT: _____

HCG DOSAGE: _____

HUNGER LEVEL: _____

BEDTIME/WAKE TIME: _____

HOURS SLEEP: _____

TOTAL CALORIES: _____

SUPPLEMENTS: _____

> Nobody can go back and start a new beginning, but anyone can start today and MAKE A NEW ENDING.
>
> - Tony Robbins

☐ Multivitamin   ☐ B12 Shot   ☐ Lipo Shot

INJECTION LOCATION   TIME: _____

☐ Belly   ☐ Deltoid   ☐ Thigh   ☐ Other: _____

DROPS / PELLETS DOSE TIMING

1st Dose: _____   2nd Dose: _____
3rd Dose: _____   4th Dose: _____

PERSONAL NOTES

....

....

....

....

....

....

....

LIQUIDS:

4	LITERS
3.5	LITERS
3	LITERS
2.5	LITERS
2	LITERS
1.5	LITERS
1	LITER
.5	LITERS

128 oz = 1 GALLON
120 oz
112 oz
104 oz
96 oz = 3 QUARTS
88 oz
80 oz
72 oz
64 oz = 2 QUARTS
56 oz
48 oz
40 oz
32 oz = 1 QUART
24 oz
16 oz
8 oz = 1 CUP

BREAKFAST   Time :

☐ None   ☐ Fruit: _____   ☐ Protein: _____   Calories: _____

Serving Size: _____   Serving Size: _____

LUNCH Time :   WAS AN ITEM EATEN AS A SNACK? WHICH?   Time:

Protein:
- ☐ Chicken breast
- ☐ Beef
- ☐ Veal
- ☐ Shrimp
- ☐ Lobster
- ☐ White fish: _____
- ☐ Protein Shake
- ☐ Other: _____

Serving Size:
- ☐ 100 grams/3.5 oz
- ☐ Other: _____

Calories: _____

Vegetable:
- ☐ Asparagus
- ☐ Beet Greens
- ☐ Cabbage
- ☐ Celery
- ☐ Chard
- ☐ Cucumber
- ☐ Fennel
- ☐ Lettuce
- ☐ Onions
- ☐ Radishes
- ☐ Spinach
- ☐ Tomatoes
- ☐ Other: _____
- ☐ Other: _____
- ☐ Other: _____

Calories: _____

Fruit:
- ☐ Strawberries
- ☐ ½ Grapefruit
- ☐ Apple
- ☐ Orange
- ☐ Other: _____

Starch:
- ☐ Grissini
- ☐ Melba
- ☐ Other: _____

Calories: _____

Other:
- ☐ TBS. Milk
- ☐ Juice of 1 Lemon
- ☐ Stevia
- ☐ Shirataki/Miracle Noodles
- ☐ Other: _____
- ☐ Other: _____
- ☐ Other: _____

Calories: _____

DINNER Time :   WAS AN ITEM EATEN AS A SNACK? WHICH?   Time:

Protein:
- ☐ Chicken
- ☐ Beef
- ☐ Veal
- ☐ Shrimp
- ☐ Lobster
- ☐ White fish: _____
- ☐ Protein Shake
- ☐ Other: _____

Serving Size:
- ☐ 100 grams
- ☐ Other: _____

Calories: _____

Vegetable:
- ☐ Asparagus
- ☐ Beet Greens
- ☐ Cabbage
- ☐ Celery
- ☐ Chard
- ☐ Cucumber
- ☐ Fennel
- ☐ Lettuce
- ☐ Onions
- ☐ Radishes
- ☐ Spinach
- ☐ Tomatoes
- ☐ Other: _____
- ☐ Other: _____
- ☐ Other: _____

Calories: _____

Fruit:
- ☐ Strawberries
- ☐ ½ Grapefruit
- ☐ Apple
- ☐ Orange
- ☐ Other: _____

Starch:
- ☐ Grissini
- ☐ Melba
- ☐ Other: _____

Calories: _____

Other:
- ☐ TBS. Milk
- ☐ Juice of 1 Lemon
- ☐ Stevia
- ☐ Shirataki/Miracle Noodles
- ☐ Other: _____
- ☐ Other: _____
- ☐ Other: _____

Calories: _____

VLCD 53 (Date): _____

WEIGHT: _____

HCG DOSAGE: _____

HUNGER LEVEL: _____

BEDTIME/WAKE TIME: _____

HOURS SLEEP: _____

TOTAL CALORIES: _____

SUPPLEMENTS: _____

☐ Multivitamin   ☐ B12 Shot   ☐ Lipo Shot

INJECTION LOCATION   TIME: _____

☐ Belly   ☐ Deltoid   ☐ Thigh   ☐ Other: _____

DROPS / PELLETS DOSE TIMING

1st Dose: _____   2nd Dose: _____

3rd Dose: _____   4th Dose: _____

PERSONAL NOTES

....
....
....
....
....
....
....

LIQUIDS:

4 LITERS	128 oz = 1 GALLON
3.5 LITERS	120 oz
3 LITERS	112 oz
2.5 LITERS	104 oz
2 LITERS	96 oz = 3 QUARTS
1.5 LITERS	88 oz
1 LITER	80 oz
.5 LITERS	72 oz
	64 oz = 2 QUARTS
	56 oz
	48 oz
	40 oz
	32 oz = 1 QUART
	24 oz
	16 oz
	8 oz = 1 CUP

BREAKFAST   Time :

☐ None   ☐ Fruit: _____   ☐ Protein: _____   Calories: _____

Serving Size: _____   Serving Size: _____

LUNCH Time :

Protein:
- [ ] Chicken breast
- [ ] Beef
- [ ] Veal
- [ ] Shrimp
- [ ] Lobster
- [ ] White fish: _____
- [ ] Protein Shake
- [ ] Other: _____

Serving Size:
- [ ] 100 grams/3.5 oz
- [ ] Other: _____

Vegetable:
- [ ] Asparagus
- [ ] Beet Greens
- [ ] Cabbage
- [ ] Celery
- [ ] Chard
- [ ] Cucumber
- [ ] Fennel
- [ ] Lettuce
- [ ] Onions
- [ ] Radishes
- [ ] Spinach
- [ ] Tomatoes
- [ ] Other: _____
- [ ] Other: _____
- [ ] Other: _____

Fruit:
- [ ] Strawberries
- [ ] ½ Grapefruit
- [ ] Apple
- [ ] Orange
- [ ] Other: _____

Starch:
- [ ] Grissini
- [ ] Melba
- [ ] Other: _____

Other:
- [ ] TBS. Milk
- [ ] Juice of 1 Lemon
- [ ] Stevia
- [ ] Shirataki/Miracle Noodles
- [ ] Other: _____
- [ ] Other: _____
- [ ] Other: _____

Calories: _____   Calories: _____   Calories: _____   Calories: _____

DINNER Time :

Protein:
- [ ] Chicken
- [ ] Beef
- [ ] Veal
- [ ] Shrimp
- [ ] Lobster
- [ ] White fish: _____
- [ ] Protein Shake
- [ ] Other: _____

Serving Size:
- [ ] 100 grams
- [ ] Other: _____

Vegetable:
- [ ] Asparagus
- [ ] Beet Greens
- [ ] Cabbage
- [ ] Celery
- [ ] Chard
- [ ] Cucumber
- [ ] Fennel
- [ ] Lettuce
- [ ] Onions
- [ ] Radishes
- [ ] Spinach
- [ ] Tomatoes
- [ ] Other: _____
- [ ] Other: _____
- [ ] Other: _____

Fruit:
- [ ] Strawberries
- [ ] ½ Grapefruit
- [ ] Apple
- [ ] Orange
- [ ] Other: _____

Starch:
- [ ] Grissini
- [ ] Melba
- [ ] Other: _____

Other:
- [ ] TBS. Milk
- [ ] Juice of 1 Lemon
- [ ] Stevia
- [ ] Shirataki/Miracle Noodles
- [ ] Other: _____
- [ ] Other: _____
- [ ] Other: _____

Calories: _____   Calories: _____   Calories: _____   Calories: _____

VLCD **54** (Date): _____

> What I like most about change is that it's a synonym for *hope*. If you are taking a risk, what you are really saying is, **I BELIEVE IN TOMORROW** and *I will be part of it.*
> - Linda Ellerbee

WEIGHT: _____

HCG DOSAGE: _____

HUNGER LEVEL: _____

BEDTIME/WAKE TIME: _____

HOURS SLEEP: _____

TOTAL CALORIES: _____

SUPPLEMENTS: _____

☐ Multivitamin ☐ B12 Shot ☐ Lipo Shot

INJECTION LOCATION   TIME: _____

☐ Belly ☐ Deltoid ☐ Thigh ☐ Other: _____

DROPS / PELLETS DOSE TIMING

1st Dose: _____ 2nd Dose: _____
3rd Dose: _____ 4th Dose: _____

PERSONAL NOTES

....

....

....

....

....

....

....

....

LIQUIDS:

4 LITERS	128 oz = 1 GALLON
3.5 LITERS	120 oz
3 LITERS	112 oz
2.5 LITERS	104 oz
2 LITERS	96 oz = 3 QUARTS
1.5 LITERS	88 oz
1 LITER	80 oz
.5 LITERS	72 oz
	64 oz = 2 QUARTS
	56 oz
	48 oz
	40 oz
	32 oz = 1 QUART
	24 oz
	16 oz
	8 oz = 1 CUP

BREAKFAST   Time: _____

☐ None ☐ Fruit: _____ ☐ Protein: _____ Calories: _____

Serving Size: _____ Serving Size: _____

LUNCH Time :

Time:

Protein:

- [ ] Chicken breast
- [ ] Beef
- [ ] Veal
- [ ] Shrimp
- [ ] Lobster
- [ ] White fish: _____
- [ ] Protein Shake
- [ ] Other: _____

Serving Size:
- [ ] 100 grams/3.5 oz
- [ ] Other: _____

Vegetable:

- [ ] Asparagus
- [ ] Beet Greens
- [ ] Cabbage
- [ ] Celery
- [ ] Chard
- [ ] Cucumber
- [ ] Fennel
- [ ] Lettuce
- [ ] Onions
- [ ] Radishes
- [ ] Spinach
- [ ] Tomatoes
- [ ] Other: _____
- [ ] Other: _____
- [ ] Other: _____

Fruit:

- [ ] Strawberries
- [ ] ½ Grapefruit
- [ ] Apple
- [ ] Orange
- [ ] Other: _____

Starch:

- [ ] Grissini
- [ ] Melba
- [ ] Other: _____

Other:

- [ ] TBS. Milk
- [ ] Juice of 1 Lemon
- [ ] Stevia
- [ ] Shirataki/Miracle Noodles
- [ ] Other: _____
- [ ] Other: _____
- [ ] Other: _____

Calories: _____   Calories: _____   Calories: _____   Calories: _____

DINNER Time :

Time:

Protein:

- [ ] Chicken
- [ ] Beef
- [ ] Veal
- [ ] Shrimp
- [ ] Lobster
- [ ] White fish: _____
- [ ] Protein Shake
- [ ] Other: _____

Serving Size:
- [ ] 100 grams
- [ ] Other: _____

Vegetable:

- [ ] Asparagus
- [ ] Beet Greens
- [ ] Cabbage
- [ ] Celery
- [ ] Chard
- [ ] Cucumber
- [ ] Fennel
- [ ] Lettuce
- [ ] Onions
- [ ] Radishes
- [ ] Spinach
- [ ] Tomatoes
- [ ] Other: _____
- [ ] Other: _____
- [ ] Other: _____

Fruit:

- [ ] Strawberries
- [ ] ½ Grapefruit
- [ ] Apple
- [ ] Orange
- [ ] Other: _____

Starch:

- [ ] Grissini
- [ ] Melba
- [ ] Other: _____

Other:

- [ ] TBS. Milk
- [ ] Juice of 1 Lemon
- [ ] Stevia
- [ ] Shirataki/Miracle Noodles
- [ ] Other: _____
- [ ] Other: _____
- [ ] Other: _____

Calories: _____   Calories: _____   Calories: _____   Calories: _____

VLCD 55 (Date): _____

WEIGHT: _____

HCG DOSAGE: _____

HUNGER LEVEL: _____

BEDTIME/WAKE TIME: _____

HOURS SLEEP: _____

TOTAL CALORIES: _____

SUPPLEMENTS: _____

☐ Multivitamin   ☐ B12 Shot   ☐ Lipo Shot

INJECTION LOCATION   TIME: _____

☐ Belly   ☐ Deltoid   ☐ Thigh   ☐ Other: _____

DROPS / PELLETS DOSE TIMING

1st Dose: _____   2nd Dose: _____

3rd Dose: _____   4th Dose: _____

PERSONAL NOTES

....
....
....
....
....
....
....

LIQUIDS:

4 LITERS	128 oz = 1 GALLON
3.5 LITERS	120 oz
3 LITERS	112 oz
2.5 LITERS	104 oz
2 LITERS	96 oz = 3 QUARTS
1.5 LITERS	88 oz
1 LITER	80 oz
.5 LITERS	72 oz
	64 oz = 2 QUARTS
	56 oz
	48 oz
	40 oz
	32 oz = 1 QUART
	24 oz
	16 oz
	8 oz = 1 CUP

BREAKFAST   Time:

☐ None   ☐ Fruit: _____   ☐ Protein: _____   Calories: _____

Serving Size: _____   Serving Size: _____

LUNCH Time :

Protein:
- [ ] Chicken breast
- [ ] Beef
- [ ] Veal
- [ ] Shrimp
- [ ] Lobster
- [ ] White fish: _____
- [ ] Protein Shake
- [ ] Other: _____

Serving Size:
- [ ] 100 grams/3.5 oz
- [ ] Other: _____

Vegetable:
- [ ] Asparagus
- [ ] Beet Greens
- [ ] Cabbage
- [ ] Celery
- [ ] Chard
- [ ] Cucumber
- [ ] Fennel
- [ ] Lettuce
- [ ] Onions
- [ ] Radishes
- [ ] Spinach
- [ ] Tomatoes
- [ ] Other: _____
- [ ] Other: _____
- [ ] Other: _____

Fruit:
- [ ] Strawberries
- [ ] ½ Grapefruit
- [ ] Apple
- [ ] Orange
- [ ] Other: _____

Starch:
- [ ] Grissini
- [ ] Melba
- [ ] Other: _____

Other:
- [ ] TBS. Milk
- [ ] Juice of 1 Lemon
- [ ] Stevia
- [ ] Shirataki/Miracle Noodles
- [ ] Other: _____
- [ ] Other: _____
- [ ] Other: _____

Calories: _____   Calories: _____   Calories: _____   Calories: _____

DINNER Time :

Protein:
- [ ] Chicken
- [ ] Beef
- [ ] Veal
- [ ] Shrimp
- [ ] Lobster
- [ ] White fish: _____
- [ ] Protein Shake
- [ ] Other: _____

Serving Size:
- [ ] 100 grams
- [ ] Other: _____

Vegetable:
- [ ] Asparagus
- [ ] Beet Greens
- [ ] Cabbage
- [ ] Celery
- [ ] Chard
- [ ] Cucumber
- [ ] Fennel
- [ ] Lettuce
- [ ] Onions
- [ ] Radishes
- [ ] Spinach
- [ ] Tomatoes
- [ ] Other: _____
- [ ] Other: _____
- [ ] Other: _____

Fruit:
- [ ] Strawberries
- [ ] ½ Grapefruit
- [ ] Apple
- [ ] Orange
- [ ] Other: _____

Starch:
- [ ] Grissini
- [ ] Melba
- [ ] Other: _____

Other:
- [ ] TBS. Milk
- [ ] Juice of 1 Lemon
- [ ] Stevia
- [ ] Shirataki/Miracle Noodles
- [ ] Other: _____
- [ ] Other: _____
- [ ] Other: _____

Calories: _____   Calories: _____   Calories: _____   Calories: _____

VLCD **56** (Date): _____

WEIGHT: _____

HCG DOSAGE: _____

HUNGER LEVEL: _____

BEDTIME/WAKE TIME: _____

HOURS SLEEP: _____

TOTAL CALORIES: _____

SUPPLEMENTS: _____

☐ Multivitamin ☐ B12 Shot ☐ Lipo Shot

> Too many people, when they make a mistake, just keep stubbornly plowing ahead and end up repeating the **SAME MISTAKES.** I believe in the motto, "Try and try again." But the way I read it, it says, **"TRY, THEN STOP AND THINK.** Then try again.
> - William Singleton

INJECTION LOCATION   TIME: _____

☐ Belly ☐ Deltoid ☐ Thigh ☐ Other: _____

DROPS / PELLETS DOSE TIMING

1st Dose: _____   2nd Dose: _____
3rd Dose: _____   4th Dose: _____

PERSONAL NOTES

....
....
....
....
....
....
....

LIQUIDS:

4 LITERS	128 oz = 1 GALLON
3.5 LITERS	120 oz
3 LITERS	112 oz
2.5 LITERS	104 oz
2 LITERS	96 oz = 3 QUARTS
1.5 LITERS	88 oz
1 LITER	80 oz
.5 LITERS	72 oz
	64 oz = 2 QUARTS
	56 oz
	48 oz
	40 oz
	32 oz = 1 QUART
	24 oz
	16 oz
	8 oz = 1 CUP

BREAKFAST   Time : _____

☐ None ☐ Fruit: _____   ☐ Protein: _____   Calories: _____
Serving Size: _____   Serving Size: _____

LUNCH Time: _____   WAS AN ITEM EATEN AS A SNACK? WHICH?   Time: _____

Protein:
- ☐ Chicken breast
- ☐ Beef
- ☐ Veal
- ☐ Shrimp
- ☐ Lobster
- ☐ White fish: _____
- ☐ Protein Shake
- ☐ Other: _____

Serving Size:
- ☐ 100 grams/3.5 oz
- ☐ Other: _____

Calories: _____

Vegetable:
- ☐ Asparagus
- ☐ Beet Greens
- ☐ Cabbage
- ☐ Celery
- ☐ Chard
- ☐ Cucumber
- ☐ Fennel
- ☐ Lettuce
- ☐ Onions
- ☐ Radishes
- ☐ Spinach
- ☐ Tomatoes
- ☐ Other: _____
- ☐ Other: _____
- ☐ Other: _____

Calories: _____

Fruit:
- ☐ Strawberries
- ☐ ½ Grapefruit
- ☐ Apple
- ☐ Orange
- ☐ Other: _____

Starch:
- ☐ Grissini
- ☐ Melba
- ☐ Other: _____

Calories: _____

Other:
- ☐ TBS. Milk
- ☐ Juice of 1 Lemon
- ☐ Stevia
- ☐ Shirataki/Miracle Noodles
- ☐ Other: _____
- ☐ Other: _____
- ☐ Other: _____

Calories: _____

DINNER Time: _____   WAS AN ITEM EATEN AS A SNACK? WHICH?   Time: _____

Protein:
- ☐ Chicken
- ☐ Beef
- ☐ Veal
- ☐ Shrimp
- ☐ Lobster
- ☐ White fish: _____
- ☐ Protein Shake
- ☐ Other: _____

Serving Size:
- ☐ 100 grams
- ☐ Other: _____

Calories: _____

Vegetable:
- ☐ Asparagus
- ☐ Beet Greens
- ☐ Cabbage
- ☐ Celery
- ☐ Chard
- ☐ Cucumber
- ☐ Fennel
- ☐ Lettuce
- ☐ Onions
- ☐ Radishes
- ☐ Spinach
- ☐ Tomatoes
- ☐ Other: _____
- ☐ Other: _____
- ☐ Other: _____

Calories: _____

Fruit:
- ☐ Strawberries
- ☐ ½ Grapefruit
- ☐ Apple
- ☐ Orange
- ☐ Other: _____

Starch:
- ☐ Grissini
- ☐ Melba
- ☐ Other: _____

Calories: _____

Other:
- ☐ TBS. Milk
- ☐ Juice of 1 Lemon
- ☐ Stevia
- ☐ Shirataki/Miracle Noodles
- ☐ Other: _____
- ☐ Other: _____
- ☐ Other: _____

Calories: _____

Reflections ON WEEK 8

REMEMBER, THIS IS NOT JUST ABOUT LOSING WEIGHT. IT'S ABOUT CHANGING YOUR WHOLE MINDSET ABOUT FOOD AND YOUR BODY,

YOU ARE BREAKING OLD PATTERNS RIGHT NOW. YOU ARE CREATING NEW PATTERNS. TRY NOT TO FOCUS YOUR PROGESS SOLELY ON WEIGHT LOSS.

SO WITH THAT IN MIND, HOW DID THIS WEEK GO?

What are you proud of? Why are you proud of it? What did you struggle with? What would you like to work on changing? What specific logical ways can you think of to make those adjustments? Or maybe you're just burned out at the moment - it's okay to just make it a rant.

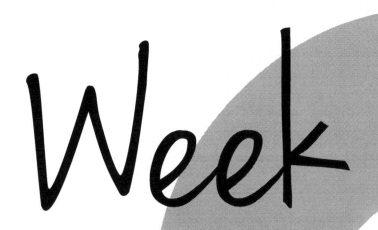

Week

9

"WE SHOULD NOT judge people by their peak of excellence, but by the distance they have traveled from the point where they started."

-Henry Ward Beecher

VLCD **57** (Date): _____

WEIGHT: _____

HCG DOSAGE: _____

HUNGER LEVEL: _____

BEDTIME/WAKE TIME: _____

HOURS SLEEP: _____

TOTAL CALORIES: _____

SUPPLEMENTS: _____

☐ Multivitamin ☐ B12 Shot ☐ Lipo Shot

INJECTION LOCATION   TIME: _____

☐ Belly ☐ Deltoid ☐ Thigh ☐ Other: _____

DROPS / PELLETS DOSE TIMING

1st Dose: _____   2nd Dose: _____

3rd Dose: _____   4th Dose: _____

PERSONAL NOTES

....

....

....

....

....

....

LIQUIDS:

4 LITERS		128 oz = 1 GALLON
3.5 LITERS		120 oz
3 LITERS		112 oz
2.5 LITERS		104 oz
2 LITERS		96 oz = 3 QUARTS
1.5 LITERS		88 oz
1 LITER		80 oz
.5 LITERS		72 oz
		64 oz = 2 QUARTS
		56 oz
		48 oz
		40 oz
		32 oz = 1 QUART
		24 oz
		16 oz
		8 oz = 1 CUP

BREAKFAST   Time :

☐ None ☐ Fruit: _____   ☐ Protein: _____   Calories: _____

Serving Size: _____   Serving Size: _____

LUNCH Time :   WAS AN ITEM EATEN AS A SNACK? WHICH?   Time:

Protein:
- [ ] Chicken breast
- [ ] Beef
- [ ] Veal
- [ ] Shrimp
- [ ] Lobster
- [ ] White fish: _____
- [ ] Protein Shake
- [ ] Other: _____

Serving Size:
- [ ] 100 grams/3.5 oz
- [ ] Other: _____

Vegetable:
- [ ] Asparagus
- [ ] Beet Greens
- [ ] Cabbage
- [ ] Celery
- [ ] Chard
- [ ] Cucumber
- [ ] Fennel
- [ ] Lettuce
- [ ] Onions
- [ ] Radishes
- [ ] Spinach
- [ ] Tomatoes
- [ ] Other: _____
- [ ] Other: _____
- [ ] Other: _____

Fruit:
- [ ] Strawberries
- [ ] ½ Grapefruit
- [ ] Apple
- [ ] Orange
- [ ] Other: _____

Starch:
- [ ] Grissini
- [ ] Melba
- [ ] Other: _____

Other:
- [ ] TBS. Milk
- [ ] Juice of 1 Lemon
- [ ] Stevia
- [ ] Shirataki/Miracle Noodles
- [ ] Other: _____
- [ ] Other: _____
- [ ] Other: _____

Calories: _____   Calories: _____   Calories: _____   Calories: _____

DINNER Time :   WAS AN ITEM EATEN AS A SNACK? WHICH?   Time:

Protein:
- [ ] Chicken
- [ ] Beef
- [ ] Veal
- [ ] Shrimp
- [ ] Lobster
- [ ] White fish: _____
- [ ] Protein Shake
- [ ] Other: _____

Serving Size:
- [ ] 100 grams
- [ ] Other: _____

Vegetable:
- [ ] Asparagus
- [ ] Beet Greens
- [ ] Cabbage
- [ ] Celery
- [ ] Chard
- [ ] Cucumber
- [ ] Fennel
- [ ] Lettuce
- [ ] Onions
- [ ] Radishes
- [ ] Spinach
- [ ] Tomatoes
- [ ] Other: _____
- [ ] Other: _____
- [ ] Other: _____

Fruit:
- [ ] Strawberries
- [ ] ½ Grapefruit
- [ ] Apple
- [ ] Orange
- [ ] Other: _____

Starch:
- [ ] Grissini
- [ ] Melba
- [ ] Other: _____

Other:
- [ ] TBS. Milk
- [ ] Juice of 1 Lemon
- [ ] Stevia
- [ ] Shirataki/Miracle Noodles
- [ ] Other: _____
- [ ] Other: _____
- [ ] Other: _____

Calories: _____   Calories: _____   Calories: _____   Calories: _____

VLCD 58 (Date): _____

WEIGHT: _____

HCG DOSAGE: _____

HUNGER LEVEL: _____

BEDTIME/WAKE TIME: _____

HOURS SLEEP: _____

TOTAL CALORIES: _____

SUPPLEMENTS: _____

☐ Multivitamin   ☐ B12 Shot   ☐ Lipo Shot

Perfect does not mean perfect actions in a perfect world, but APPROPRIATE ACTIONS in an imperfect one.
- R.H. Blyth

INJECTION LOCATION   TIME: _____

☐ Belly   ☐ Deltoid   ☐ Thigh   ☐ Other: _____

DROPS / PELLETS DOSE TIMING

1st Dose: _____   2nd Dose: _____

3rd Dose: _____   4th Dose: _____

PERSONAL NOTES

....
....
....
....
....
....
....
....

LIQUIDS:

4 LITERS	128 oz = 1 GALLON
3.5 LITERS	120 oz
3 LITERS	112 oz
2.5 LITERS	104 oz
2 LITERS	96 oz = 3 QUARTS
1.5 LITERS	88 oz
1 LITER	80 oz
.5 LITERS	72 oz
	64 oz = 2 QUARTS
	56 oz
	48 oz
	40 oz
	32 oz = 1 QUART
	24 oz
	16 oz
	8 oz = 1 CUP

BREAKFAST   Time : _____

☐ None   ☐ Fruit: _____   ☐ Protein: _____   Calories: _____

Serving Size: _____   Serving Size: _____

LUNCH Time :   WAS AN ITEM EATEN AS A SNACK? WHICH?   Time:

Protein:
- ☐ Chicken breast
- ☐ Beef
- ☐ Veal
- ☐ Shrimp
- ☐ Lobster
- ☐ White fish: _____
- ☐ Protein Shake
- ☐ Other: _____

Serving Size:
- ☐ 100 grams/3.5 oz
- ☐ Other: _____

Vegetable:
- ☐ Asparagus
- ☐ Beet Greens
- ☐ Cabbage
- ☐ Celery
- ☐ Chard
- ☐ Cucumber
- ☐ Fennel
- ☐ Lettuce
- ☐ Onions
- ☐ Radishes
- ☐ Spinach
- ☐ Tomatoes
- ☐ Other: _____
- ☐ Other: _____
- ☐ Other: _____

Fruit:
- ☐ Strawberries
- ☐ ½ Grapefruit
- ☐ Apple
- ☐ Orange
- ☐ Other: _____

Starch:
- ☐ Grissini
- ☐ Melba
- ☐ Other: _____

Other:
- ☐ TBS. Milk
- ☐ Juice of 1 Lemon
- ☐ Stevia
- ☐ Shirataki/Miracle Noodles
- ☐ Other: _____
- ☐ Other: _____
- ☐ Other: _____

Calories: _____ Calories: _____ Calories: _____ Calories: _____

DINNER Time :   WAS AN ITEM EATEN AS A SNACK? WHICH?   Time:

Protein:
- ☐ Chicken
- ☐ Beef
- ☐ Veal
- ☐ Shrimp
- ☐ Lobster
- ☐ White fish: _____
- ☐ Protein Shake
- ☐ Other: _____

Serving Size:
- ☐ 100 grams
- ☐ Other: _____

Vegetable:
- ☐ Asparagus
- ☐ Beet Greens
- ☐ Cabbage
- ☐ Celery
- ☐ Chard
- ☐ Cucumber
- ☐ Fennel
- ☐ Lettuce
- ☐ Onions
- ☐ Radishes
- ☐ Spinach
- ☐ Tomatoes
- ☐ Other: _____
- ☐ Other: _____
- ☐ Other: _____

Fruit:
- ☐ Strawberries
- ☐ ½ Grapefruit
- ☐ Apple
- ☐ Orange
- ☐ Other: _____

Starch:
- ☐ Grissini
- ☐ Melba
- ☐ Other: _____

Other:
- ☐ TBS. Milk
- ☐ Juice of 1 Lemon
- ☐ Stevia
- ☐ Shirataki/Miracle Noodles
- ☐ Other: _____
- ☐ Other: _____
- ☐ Other: _____

Calories: _____ Calories: _____ Calories: _____ Calories: _____

VLCD **59** (Date): _____

WEIGHT: _____

HCG DOSAGE: _____

HUNGER LEVEL: _____

BEDTIME/WAKE TIME: _____

HOURS SLEEP: _____

TOTAL CALORIES: _____

SUPPLEMENTS: _____

☐ Multivitamin ☐ B12 Shot ☐ Lipo Shot

INJECTION LOCATION TIME: _____

☐ Belly ☐ Deltoid ☐ Thigh ☐ Other: _____

DROPS / PELLETS DOSE TIMING

1st Dose: _____   2nd Dose: _____
3rd Dose: _____   4th Dose: _____

LIQUIDS:

4 LITERS	128 oz = 1 GALLON
3.5 LITERS	120 oz
3 LITERS	112 oz
2.5 LITERS	104 oz
2 LITERS	96 oz = 3 QUARTS
1.5 LITERS	88 oz
1 LITER	80 oz
.5 LITERS	72 oz
	64 oz = 2 QUARTS
	56 oz
	48 oz
	40 oz
	32 oz = 1 QUART
	24 oz
	16 oz
	8 oz = 1 CUP

PERSONAL NOTES

....

....

....

....

....

....

BREAKFAST   Time:

☐ None ☐ Fruit: _____   ☐ Protein: _____   Calories: _____
        Serving Size: _____   Serving Size: _____

LUNCH Time :   WAS AN ITEM EATEN AS A SNACK? WHICH?   Time:

Protein:
- ☐ Chicken breast
- ☐ Beef
- ☐ Veal
- ☐ Shrimp
- ☐ Lobster
- ☐ White fish: _____
- ☐ Protein Shake
- ☐ Other: _____

Serving Size:
- ☐ 100 grams/3.5 oz
- ☐ Other: _____

Vegetable:
- ☐ Asparagus
- ☐ Beet Greens
- ☐ Cabbage
- ☐ Celery
- ☐ Chard
- ☐ Cucumber
- ☐ Fennel
- ☐ Lettuce
- ☐ Onions
- ☐ Radishes
- ☐ Spinach
- ☐ Tomatoes
- ☐ Other: _____
- ☐ Other: _____
- ☐ Other: _____

Fruit:
- ☐ Strawberries
- ☐ ½ Grapefruit
- ☐ Apple
- ☐ Orange
- ☐ Other: _____

Starch:
- ☐ Grissini
- ☐ Melba
- ☐ Other: _____

Other:
- ☐ TBS. Milk
- ☐ Juice of 1 Lemon
- ☐ Stevia
- ☐ Shirataki/Miracle Noodles
- ☐ Other: _____
- ☐ Other: _____
- ☐ Other: _____

Calories: _____   Calories: _____   Calories: _____   Calories: _____

DINNER Time :   WAS AN ITEM EATEN AS A SNACK? WHICH?   Time:

Protein:
- ☐ Chicken
- ☐ Beef
- ☐ Veal
- ☐ Shrimp
- ☐ Lobster
- ☐ White fish: _____
- ☐ Protein Shake
- ☐ Other: _____

Serving Size:
- ☐ 100 grams
- ☐ Other: _____

Vegetable:
- ☐ Asparagus
- ☐ Beet Greens
- ☐ Cabbage
- ☐ Celery
- ☐ Chard
- ☐ Cucumber
- ☐ Fennel
- ☐ Lettuce
- ☐ Onions
- ☐ Radishes
- ☐ Spinach
- ☐ Tomatoes
- ☐ Other: _____
- ☐ Other: _____
- ☐ Other: _____

Fruit:
- ☐ Strawberries
- ☐ ½ Grapefruit
- ☐ Apple
- ☐ Orange
- ☐ Other: _____

Starch:
- ☐ Grissini
- ☐ Melba
- ☐ Other: _____

Other:
- ☐ TBS. Milk
- ☐ Juice of 1 Lemon
- ☐ Stevia
- ☐ Shirataki/Miracle Noodles
- ☐ Other: _____
- ☐ Other: _____
- ☐ Other: _____

Calories: _____   Calories: _____   Calories: _____   Calories: _____

VLCD **60** (Date): _____

> If you are going to *doubt* something, DOUBT YOUR LIMITS.
>
> *- Don Ward*

WEIGHT: _____

HCG DOSAGE: _____

HUNGER LEVEL: _____

BEDTIME/WAKE TIME: _____

HOURS SLEEP: _____

TOTAL CALORIES: _____

SUPPLEMENTS: _____

☐ Multivitamin   ☐ B12 Shot   ☐ Lipo Shot

INJECTION LOCATION   TIME: _____

☐ Belly   ☐ Deltoid   ☐ Thigh   ☐ Other: _____

DROPS / PELLETS DOSE TIMING

1st Dose: _____   2nd Dose: _____

3rd Dose: _____   4th Dose: _____

PERSONAL NOTES

....

....

....

....

....

....

....

LIQUIDS:

4 LITERS		128 oz = 1 GALLON
3.5 LITERS		120 oz
3 LITERS		112 oz
2.5 LITERS		104 oz
2 LITERS		96 oz = 3 QUARTS
1.5 LITERS		88 oz
1 LITER		80 oz
.5 LITERS		72 oz
		64 oz = 2 QUARTS
		56 oz
		48 oz
		40 oz
		32 oz = 1 QUART
		24 oz
		16 oz
		8 oz = 1 CUP

BREAKFAST   Time : _____

....

☐ None   ☐ Fruit: _____   ☐ Protein: _____   *Calories:* _____

   Serving Size: _____   *Serving Size:* _____

LUNCH Time :   WAS AN ITEM EATEN AS A SNACK? WHICH?   Time:

Protein:
- ☐ Chicken breast
- ☐ Beef
- ☐ Veal
- ☐ Shrimp
- ☐ Lobster
- ☐ White fish: _____
- ☐ Protein Shake
- ☐ Other: _____

Serving Size:
- ☐ 100 grams/3.5 oz
- ☐ Other: _____

Vegetable:
- ☐ Asparagus
- ☐ Beet Greens
- ☐ Cabbage
- ☐ Celery
- ☐ Chard
- ☐ Cucumber
- ☐ Fennel
- ☐ Lettuce
- ☐ Onions
- ☐ Radishes
- ☐ Spinach
- ☐ Tomatoes
- ☐ Other: _____
- ☐ Other: _____
- ☐ Other: _____

Fruit:
- ☐ Strawberries
- ☐ ½ Grapefruit
- ☐ Apple
- ☐ Orange
- ☐ Other: _____

Starch:
- ☐ Grissini
- ☐ Melba
- ☐ Other: _____

Other:
- ☐ TBS. Milk
- ☐ Juice of 1 Lemon
- ☐ Stevia
- ☐ Shirataki/Miracle Noodles
- ☐ Other: _____
- ☐ Other: _____
- ☐ Other: _____

Calories: _____   Calories: _____   Calories: _____   Calories: _____

DINNER Time :   WAS AN ITEM EATEN AS A SNACK? WHICH?   Time:

Protein:
- ☐ Chicken
- ☐ Beef
- ☐ Veal
- ☐ Shrimp
- ☐ Lobster
- ☐ White fish: _____
- ☐ Protein Shake
- ☐ Other: _____

Serving Size:
- ☐ 100 grams
- ☐ Other: _____

Vegetable:
- ☐ Asparagus
- ☐ Beet Greens
- ☐ Cabbage
- ☐ Celery
- ☐ Chard
- ☐ Cucumber
- ☐ Fennel
- ☐ Lettuce
- ☐ Onions
- ☐ Radishes
- ☐ Spinach
- ☐ Tomatoes
- ☐ Other: _____
- ☐ Other: _____
- ☐ Other: _____

Fruit:
- ☐ Strawberries
- ☐ ½ Grapefruit
- ☐ Apple
- ☐ Orange
- ☐ Other: _____

Starch:
- ☐ Grissini
- ☐ Melba
- ☐ Other: _____

Other:
- ☐ TBS. Milk
- ☐ Juice of 1 Lemon
- ☐ Stevia
- ☐ Shirataki/Miracle Noodles
- ☐ Other: _____
- ☐ Other: _____
- ☐ Other: _____

Calories: _____   Calories: _____   Calories: _____   Calories: _____

VLCD **61** (Date): _____

WEIGHT: _____

HCG DOSAGE: _____

HUNGER LEVEL: _____

BEDTIME/WAKE TIME: _____

HOURS SLEEP: _____

TOTAL CALORIES: _____

SUPPLEMENTS: _____

☐ Multivitamin ☐ B12 Shot ☐ Lipo Shot

INJECTION LOCATION   TIME: _____

☐ Belly ☐ Deltoid ☐ Thigh ☐ Other: _____

DROPS / PELLETS DOSE TIMING

1st Dose: _____   2nd Dose: _____

3rd Dose: _____   4th Dose: _____

PERSONAL NOTES

....
....
....
....
....
....
....

LIQUIDS:

4 LITERS	128 oz = 1 GALLON
3.5 LITERS	120 oz
3 LITERS	112 oz
2.5 LITERS	104 oz
2 LITERS	96 oz = 3 QUARTS
1.5 LITERS	88 oz
1 LITER	80 oz
.5 LITERS	72 oz
	64 oz = 2 QUARTS
	56 oz
	48 oz
	40 oz
	32 oz = 1 QUART
	24 oz
	16 oz
	8 oz = 1 CUP

BREAKFAST   Time :

☐ None ☐ Fruit: _____   ☐ Protein: _____   Calories: _____

Serving Size: _____   Serving Size: _____

LUNCH Time: WAS AN ITEM EATEN AS A SNACK? WHICH?   Time:

Protein:
- ☐ Chicken breast
- ☐ Beef
- ☐ Veal
- ☐ Shrimp
- ☐ Lobster
- ☐ White fish: _____
- ☐ Protein Shake
- ☐ Other: _____

Serving Size:
- ☐ 100 grams/3.5 oz
- ☐ Other: _____

Vegetable:
- ☐ Asparagus
- ☐ Beet Greens
- ☐ Cabbage
- ☐ Celery
- ☐ Chard
- ☐ Cucumber
- ☐ Fennel
- ☐ Lettuce
- ☐ Onions
- ☐ Radishes
- ☐ Spinach
- ☐ Tomatoes
- ☐ Other: _____
- ☐ Other: _____
- ☐ Other: _____

Fruit:
- ☐ Strawberries
- ☐ ½ Grapefruit
- ☐ Apple
- ☐ Orange
- ☐ Other: _____

Starch:
- ☐ Grissini
- ☐ Melba
- ☐ Other: _____

Other:
- ☐ TBS. Milk
- ☐ Juice of 1 Lemon
- ☐ Stevia
- ☐ Shirataki/Miracle Noodles
- ☐ Other: _____
- ☐ Other: _____
- ☐ Other: _____

Calories: _____   Calories: _____   Calories: _____   Calories: _____

DINNER Time: WAS AN ITEM EATEN AS A SNACK? WHICH?   Time:

Protein:
- ☐ Chicken
- ☐ Beef
- ☐ Veal
- ☐ Shrimp
- ☐ Lobster
- ☐ White fish: _____
- ☐ Protein Shake
- ☐ Other: _____

Serving Size:
- ☐ 100 grams
- ☐ Other: _____

Vegetable:
- ☐ Asparagus
- ☐ Beet Greens
- ☐ Cabbage
- ☐ Celery
- ☐ Chard
- ☐ Cucumber
- ☐ Fennel
- ☐ Lettuce
- ☐ Onions
- ☐ Radishes
- ☐ Spinach
- ☐ Tomatoes
- ☐ Other: _____
- ☐ Other: _____
- ☐ Other: _____

Fruit:
- ☐ Strawberries
- ☐ ½ Grapefruit
- ☐ Apple
- ☐ Orange
- ☐ Other: _____

Starch:
- ☐ Grissini
- ☐ Melba
- ☐ Other: _____

Other:
- ☐ TBS. Milk
- ☐ Juice of 1 Lemon
- ☐ Stevia
- ☐ Shirataki/Miracle Noodles
- ☐ Other: _____
- ☐ Other: _____
- ☐ Other: _____

Calories: _____   Calories: _____   Calories: _____   Calories: _____

VLCD 62 (Date): _____

WEIGHT: _____

HCG DOSAGE: _____

HUNGER LEVEL: _____

BEDTIME/WAKE TIME: _____

HOURS SLEEP: _____

TOTAL CALORIES: _____

SUPPLEMENTS: _____

☐ Multivitamin   ☐ B12 Shot   ☐ Lipo Shot

"DON'T SPEND TIME BEATING ON A WALL, HOPING TO TRANSFORM IT INTO A DOOR."
- Coco Chanel

INJECTION LOCATION   TIME: _____

☐ Belly   ☐ Deltoid   ☐ Thigh   ☐ Other: _____

DROPS / PELLETS DOSE TIMING

1st Dose: _____   2nd Dose: _____

3rd Dose: _____   4th Dose: _____

PERSONAL NOTES

....
....
....
....
....
....
....

LIQUIDS:

4 LITERS	
3.5 LITERS	
3 LITERS	
2.5 LITERS	
2 LITERS	
1.5 LITERS	
1 LITER	
.5 LITERS	

128 oz = 1 GALLON	
120 oz	
112 oz	
104 oz	
96 oz = 3 QUARTS	
88 oz	
80 oz	
72 oz	
64 oz = 2 QUARTS	
56 oz	
48 oz	
40 oz	
32 oz = 1 QUART	
24 oz	
16 oz	
8 oz = 1 CUP	

BREAKFAST   Time :

☐ None   ☐ Fruit: _____   ☐ Protein: _____   Calories: _____

Serving Size: _____   Serving Size: _____

LUNCH Time :

Protein:
- ☐ Chicken breast
- ☐ Beef
- ☐ Veal
- ☐ Shrimp
- ☐ Lobster
- ☐ White fish: _____
- ☐ Protein Shake
- ☐ Other: _____

Serving Size:
- ☐ 100 grams/3.5 oz
- ☐ Other: _____

Vegetable:
- ☐ Asparagus
- ☐ Beet Greens
- ☐ Cabbage
- ☐ Celery
- ☐ Chard
- ☐ Cucumber
- ☐ Fennel
- ☐ Lettuce
- ☐ Onions
- ☐ Radishes
- ☐ Spinach
- ☐ Tomatoes
- ☐ Other: _____
- ☐ Other: _____
- ☐ Other: _____

Fruit:
- ☐ Strawberries
- ☐ ½ Grapefruit
- ☐ Apple
- ☐ Orange
- ☐ Other: _____

Starch:
- ☐ Grissini
- ☐ Melba
- ☐ Other: _____

Other:
- ☐ TBS. Milk
- ☐ Juice of 1 Lemon
- ☐ Stevia
- ☐ Shirataki/Miracle Noodles
- ☐ Other: _____
- ☐ Other: _____
- ☐ Other: _____

Calories: _____   Calories: _____   Calories: _____   Calories: _____

DINNER Time :

Protein:
- ☐ Chicken
- ☐ Beef
- ☐ Veal
- ☐ Shrimp
- ☐ Lobster
- ☐ White fish: _____
- ☐ Protein Shake
- ☐ Other: _____

Serving Size:
- ☐ 100 grams
- ☐ Other: _____

Vegetable:
- ☐ Asparagus
- ☐ Beet Greens
- ☐ Cabbage
- ☐ Celery
- ☐ Chard
- ☐ Cucumber
- ☐ Fennel
- ☐ Lettuce
- ☐ Onions
- ☐ Radishes
- ☐ Spinach
- ☐ Tomatoes
- ☐ Other: _____
- ☐ Other: _____
- ☐ Other: _____

Fruit:
- ☐ Strawberries
- ☐ ½ Grapefruit
- ☐ Apple
- ☐ Orange
- ☐ Other: _____

Starch:
- ☐ Grissini
- ☐ Melba
- ☐ Other: _____

Other:
- ☐ TBS. Milk
- ☐ Juice of 1 Lemon
- ☐ Stevia
- ☐ Shirataki/Miracle Noodles
- ☐ Other: _____
- ☐ Other: _____
- ☐ Other: _____

Calories: _____   Calories: _____   Calories: _____   Calories: _____

VLCD 63 (Date): _____

WEIGHT: _____

HCG DOSAGE: _____

HUNGER LEVEL: _____

BEDTIME/WAKE TIME: _____

HOURS SLEEP: _____

TOTAL CALORIES: _____

SUPPLEMENTS: _____

☐ Multivitamin   ☐ B12 Shot   ☐ Lipo Shot

INJECTION LOCATION   TIME: _____

☐ Belly   ☐ Deltoid   ☐ Thigh   ☐ Other: _____

DROPS / PELLETS DOSE TIMING

1st Dose: _____   2nd Dose: _____

3rd Dose: _____   4th Dose: _____

PERSONAL NOTES

....

....

....

....

....

....

....

....

LIQUIDS:

4 LITERS		128 oz = 1 GALLON
3.5 LITERS		120 oz
3 LITERS		112 oz
2.5 LITERS		104 oz
2 LITERS		96 oz = 3 QUARTS
1.5 LITERS		88 oz
1 LITER		80 oz
.5 LITERS		72 oz
		64 oz = 2 QUARTS
		56 oz
		48 oz
		40 oz
		32 oz = 1 QUART
		24 oz
		16 oz
		8 oz = 1 CUP

BREAKFAST   Time :

☐ None   ☐ Fruit: _____   ☐ Protein: _____   Calories: _____

Serving Size: _____   Serving Size: _____

LUNCH Time : ____ WAS AN ITEM EATEN AS A SNACK? WHICH? Time: ____

Protein:
- [ ] Chicken breast
- [ ] Beef
- [ ] Veal
- [ ] Shrimp
- [ ] Lobster
- [ ] White fish: _____
- [ ] Protein Shake
- [ ] Other: _____

Serving Size:
- [ ] 100 grams/3.5 oz
- [ ] Other: _____

Vegetable:
- [ ] Asparagus
- [ ] Beet Greens
- [ ] Cabbage
- [ ] Celery
- [ ] Chard
- [ ] Cucumber
- [ ] Fennel
- [ ] Lettuce
- [ ] Onions
- [ ] Radishes
- [ ] Spinach
- [ ] Tomatoes
- [ ] Other: _____
- [ ] Other: _____
- [ ] Other: _____

Fruit:
- [ ] Strawberries
- [ ] ½ Grapefruit
- [ ] Apple
- [ ] Orange
- [ ] Other: _____

Starch:
- [ ] Grissini
- [ ] Melba
- [ ] Other: _____

Other:
- [ ] TBS. Milk
- [ ] Juice of 1 Lemon
- [ ] Stevia
- [ ] Shirataki/Miracle Noodles
- [ ] Other: _____
- [ ] Other: _____
- [ ] Other: _____

Calories: _____ Calories: _____ Calories: _____ Calories: _____

DINNER Time : ____ WAS AN ITEM EATEN AS A SNACK? WHICH? Time: ____

Protein:
- [ ] Chicken
- [ ] Beef
- [ ] Veal
- [ ] Shrimp
- [ ] Lobster
- [ ] White fish: _____
- [ ] Protein Shake
- [ ] Other: _____

Serving Size:
- [ ] 100 grams
- [ ] Other: _____

Vegetable:
- [ ] Asparagus
- [ ] Beet Greens
- [ ] Cabbage
- [ ] Celery
- [ ] Chard
- [ ] Cucumber
- [ ] Fennel
- [ ] Lettuce
- [ ] Onions
- [ ] Radishes
- [ ] Spinach
- [ ] Tomatoes
- [ ] Other: _____
- [ ] Other: _____
- [ ] Other: _____

Fruit:
- [ ] Strawberries
- [ ] ½ Grapefruit
- [ ] Apple
- [ ] Orange
- [ ] Other: _____

Starch:
- [ ] Grissini
- [ ] Melba
- [ ] Other: _____

Other:
- [ ] TBS. Milk
- [ ] Juice of 1 Lemon
- [ ] Stevia
- [ ] Shirataki/Miracle Noodles
- [ ] Other: _____
- [ ] Other: _____
- [ ] Other: _____

Calories: _____ Calories: _____ Calories: _____ Calories: _____

Reflections ON WEEK 9

REMEMBER, THIS IS NOT JUST ABOUT LOSING WEIGHT. IT'S ABOUT CHANGING YOUR WHOLE MINDSET ABOUT FOOD AND YOUR BODY.

YOU ARE BREAKING OLD PATTERNS RIGHT NOW. YOU ARE CREATING NEW PATTERNS. TRY NOT TO FOCUS YOUR PROGESS SOLELY ON WEIGHT LOSS.

SO WITH THAT IN MIND, HOW DID THIS WEEK GO?

What are you proud of? Why are you proud of it? What did you struggle with? What would you like to work on changing? What specific logical ways can you think of to make those adjustments? Or maybe you're just burned out at the moment - it's okay to just make it a rant.

Section

5

....

REFLECTIONS and NOTES

Reflections ON THIS ROUND

WRITE DOWN 1 MAJOR BREAKTHROUGH YOU HAD.
Breakthrough:

WHAT DID YOU LEARN ABOUT YOURSELF?
Learned:

Reflections ON THIS ROUND

WHAT DO YOU THINK IS THE CAUSE OF ANY STRUGGLES YOU EXPERIENCED? WHAT DO YOU THINK COULD PREVENT THEM NEXT TIME?

Preventing Struggles: ....

....

....

....

....

....

....

....

....

....

....

....

....

....

....

....

....

....

....

....

SETTING A GOAL IS NOT THE MAIN THING. IT IS DECIDING HOW YOU WILL GO ABOUT ACHIEVING IT AND STAYING WITH THAT PLAN.

— Tom Landry

It's time for Phase 3 isn't it?

Remember, no need to panic. Gather information so you know what to expect and can form your own personal plan.

Free resource: hcgchica.com/p3

Paid resource: P3 & P4 Workbook at

hcgchica.com/p3workbook

My NOTES

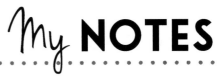

My NOTES

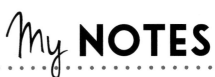

My NOTES

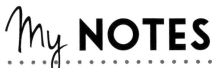

My NOTES

My NOTES

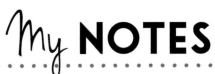

My NOTES

My NOTES

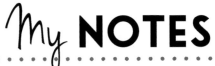

Section

6

· · · · ·

Phase 2

CALORIE

COUNT

CHARTS

A Few Thoughts on CALORIE COUNTING

To be honest, I was a little hesitant to put these calorie charts in here. My fear is that it will encourage you to over-analyze the process. I don't really care for counting calories.

Dr. Simeons designed this protocol to be simple. Twice a day, 100 grams of protein, the only food that's weighed. One fruit from the list, one veggie, no specific amount, from the list. Done. Move on with your life. Do stuff with your time that doesn't have to do with food, like children do.

25 or 50 calories here and there is not going to be the difference between you losing an extra 10 lbs on a round of hCG. There's 35,000 calories worth in ten pounds of fat, if it helps to think of it that way.

> THERE IS ONE BIG REASON THAT I LOVE THE HCG DIET'S SIMPLICITY – IT HELPS YOU GET AWAY FROM OBSESSION WITH EATING AND FOOD.

One of the most important takeaways to learn from this protocol is for life to *not* be about food. Spending too much time counting and cataloguing everything can work against this mind shift that needs to take place.

A GOOD USE for this list

So this is more what I'm hoping you'll use this list for - **something you just glance at here and there to help you make choices and have some general head knowledge of what you're consuming each day.**

If you find all the details overwhelming, forget them!

You really can't go wrong by just following the basics of Dr. Simeon's protocol which only required measuring your meat and that's it.

PROTEIN – Various Serving Sizes

You'll notice that I have a variety of portion sizes listed with the meats. There are 2 reasons for this.

One, even though the original protocol lists 100 grams across the board as the portion size to be used, there are some cases where a person may be obliged to eat an additional 3rd serving of protein, or may choose to eat a larger portion of a lower calorie per ounce meat (ie. shrimp).

There were days as I got leaner that I found I needed more than 500 calories. Robin Woodall's book *Weight Loss Apocalypse, Emotional Rehab Through the hCG Protocol*, (check out my video review of this book at hcgchica.com/hcgbooks) noted that those who were getting leaner and did not have as much weight left to lose may feel more hunger than those who are heavier. She mentioned that this may be due to the hCG hormone not being able to stimulate enough leptin to produce the same satiated effect that those who are more overweight usually experience.

When this happens, sometimes a person might choose as part of their own personal protocol to eat an additional 50 gram serving of protein for breakfast, or after a workout. Someone who is working strange work shifts with long hours may have such for a late night snack.

Additionally, those who continue to have a fairly rigorous workout regimen seem to need additional protein to prevent muscle loss.

Also useful in having these stats is that you can see there are differences in the fat content of various meats. If you end up choosing to have a larger portion of meat, say 150 grams instead of 100 grams,

A Few Thoughts on CALORIE COUNTING

you might decide to choose a lower fat protein since we are avoiding fat as much as possible.

ORIGINAL DIET
& Optional Modifications

I've added a few food choices to the calorie charts that are not on the original protocol. It is your call whether you try them. I am just putting this here because some have chosen to use these other foods with seeming success, and this makes it easy for such ones to use this workbook. **I have clearly noted what is not on the original protocol for those who wish to stick with Dr. Simeons original method.**

I have rounded off the grams and calories so we don't have a bunch of messy decimals. And lastly, some of these can't be *exact*. For instance, there is a varying amount of fat from one piece of london broil to another, but overall it is considered an extra lean cut of beef, and this will give you a good estimate of what it contains.

Quick Glance MACRO BREAKDOWN

Fruits

	SERVING SIZE INCHES	CALORIES	GRAMS SUGAR	GRAMS FIBER
APPLE SMALL	2.75	80	16	4
MEDIUM	3	93	19	4
LARGE	3.3	120	24	6
ORANGE SMALL	2.4	45	9	2
MEDIUM	2.6	62	12	3
LARGE	3.1	86	17	4
STRAWBERRIES 1/2 CUP		25	3.5	1.5
1 CUP		49	7	3
1.5 CUPS		75	10.5	4.5
1/2 GRAPEFRUIT 1/2 MED		41	9	2
1/2 LARGE		53	11	2
OTHER:				
OTHER:				

Quick Glance MACRO BREAKDOWN

Info below based on meat being weighed raw.

Beef

	SERVING SIZE		CALORIES	GRAMS PROTEIN	GRAMS FAT
	GRAMS	OZ			
95% FAT FREE GROUND BEEF	50	1.7	68	11	3
	100	3.5	136	21	5
	150	5.2	204	32	8
LONDON BROIL	50	1.7	61	11	2
	100	3.5	123	21	4
	150	5.2	184	32	5
TOP SIRLOIN STEAK	50	1.7	68	11	2
	100	3.5	136	23	4
	150	5.2	204	34	6
OTHER:					
OTHER:					
OTHER:					
VEAL, GROUND	50	1.7	72	10	3
	100	3.5	144	19	7
	150	5.2	216	29	10
VEAL, LOIN, LEAN	50	1.7	58	10	2
	100	3.5	116	20	3
	150	5.2	174	30	5
VEAL, SIRLOIN, LEAN	50	1.7	55	10	1
	100	3.5	110	20	3
	150	5.2	165	30	4

Quick Glance MACRO BREAKDOWN

Chicken & Other

	SERVING SIZE GRAMS OZ		CALORIES	GRAMS PROTEIN	GRAMS FAT
CHICKEN BREAST	50	1.7	55	12	0.6
	100	3.5	110	23	1
	150	5.2	165	35	2
1 EGG + 3 EGG WHITES			123	17	5
EGG WHITES	50	1.7	26	5	0
	100	3.5	52	11	0
	150	5.2	78	16	0
COTTAGE CHEESE FAT FREE	50	1.7	36	5	0
	100	3.5	72	10	0
	150	5.2	108	15	0
OTHER:					
OTHER:					
OTHER:					
OTHER:					
OTHER:					

Quick Glance MACRO BREAKDOWN

Seafood

	SERVING SIZE		CALORIES	GRAMS PROTEIN	GRAMS FAT
	GRAMS	OZ			
CATFISH, FARMED	50	1.7	67	8	4
	100	3.5	135	16	8
	150	5.2	202	24	12
CATFISH, WILD	50	1.7	48	8	1
	100	3.5	95	16	3
	150	5.2	143	25	4
COD	50	1.7	41	9	0
	100	3.5	82	18	1
	150	5.2	123	27	1
CRAB CANNED, DRAINED	50	1.7	42	9	0
	100	3.5	83	18	1
	150	5.2	125	27	1
FLOUNDER	50	1.7	35	6	1
	100	3.5	70	12	2
	150	5.2	105	18	2.5
HALIBUT	50	1.7	55	10	1
	100	3.5	110	21	2
	150	5.2	165	31	3
LOBSTER	50	1.7	45	9	0
	100	3.5	90	19	1
	150	5.2	135	28	1
RED SNAPPER	50	1.7	45	9.5	0
	100	3.5	89	19	1
	150	5.2	134	28	1.6
SEA BASS	50	1.7	49	9	1
	100	3.5	97	18	2
	150	5.2	146	28	3

Quick Glance MACRO BREAKDOWN

Seafood

	SERVING SIZE GRAMS OZ		CALORIES	GRAMS PROTEIN	GRAMS FAT
SHRIMP, WITH SHELL	50	1.7	35	7	0
	100	3.5	70	14	1
	150	5.2	105	21	2
SHRIMP, WITHOUT SHELL	50	1.7	53	10	1
	100	3.5	106	20	2
	150	5.2	159	30	3
SOLE	50	1.7	45	9	0
	100	3.5	89	18	1
	150	5.2	137	27	1.5
TILAPIA	50	1.7	48	10	1
	100	3.5	96	20	2
	150	5.2	144	30	3
TROUT, SKINLESS	50	1.7	47	8	1
	100	3.5	94	16	2
	150	5.2	141	24	3

Quick Glance MACRO BREAKDOWN

OFF PROTOCOL Proteins	SERVING SIZE		CALORIES	GRAMS PROTEIN	GRAMS FAT
	GRAMS	OZ			
97% FAT FREE HAM	50	1.7	54	8	2
	100	3.5	107	16	4
	150	5.2	161	24	5
99% FAT FREE GROUND TURKEY	50	1.7	56	12	1
	100	3.5	112	24	2
	150	5.2	168	35	3
WATER PACKED TUNA	50	1.7	64	12	2
	100	3.5	128	24	3
	150	5.2	192	35	4
OTHER:					
OTHER:					
OTHER:					

Quick Glance MACRO BREAKDOWN

Veggies

	SERVING SIZE	CALORIES	GRAMS TOTAL CARBS	GRAMS FIBER	NET CARBS
ASPARAGUS	1/2 CUP	14	3	1	1
	1 CUP	27	5	3	2
	1.5 CUPS	41	8	4	4
	2 CUPS	54	10	6	5
BEET GREENS	1/2 CUP	4	1	1	0
	1 CUP	8	2	1	0
	1.5 CUPS	12	2	2	0
	2 CUPS	16	3	3	0
CABBAGE	1/2 CUP	11	3	1	2
	1 CUP	22	5	2	3
	1.5 CUPS	33	8	3	5
	2 CUPS	44	10	4	6
CABBAGE, NAPA	1/2 CUP	6	1	0	1
	1 CUP	12	3	1	2
	1.5 CUPS	18	4	1	2
	2 CUPS	24	5	2	3
CABBAGE, RED	1/2 CUP	14	3	1	2
	1 CUP	28	7	2	5
	1.5 CUPS	42	10	3	7
	2 CUPS	56	13	4	9
CELERY	1/2 CUP	8	2	1	1
	1 CUP	16	3	2	1
	1.5 CUPS	24	5	2	2
	2 CUPS	32	6	3	3
CHARD	1/2 CUP	4	7	0	0
	1 CUP	7	1	1	1
	1.5 CUPS	11	2	1	1
	2 CUPS	14	3	1	1

Quick Glance MACRO BREAKDOWN

Veggies

	SERVING SIZE	CALORIES	GRAMS TOTAL CARBS	GRAMS FIBER	NET CARBS
CUCUMBER, PEELED	1/2 CUP	7	1	0	1
	1 CUP	14	3	2	2
	1.5 CUPS	21	4	1	3
	2 CUPS	28	5	2	3
CUCUMBER, WITH PEEL	1/2 CUP	8	2	0	2
	1 CUP	16	4	0	3
	1.5 CUPS	24	6	1	4
	2 CUPS	32	8	1	6
FENNEL	1/2 CUP	14	3	1	2
	1 CUP	27	6	3	4
	1.5 CUPS	41	9	4	5
	2 CUPS	54	13	5	7
LETTUCE, ROMAINE & ICEBERG	1/2 CUP	4	1	1	0
	1 CUP	8	2	1	1
	1.5 CUPS	12	2	2	1
	2 CUPS	16	3	2	1
LETTUCE, RED & GREEN LEAF	1/2 CUP	3	0	0	0
	1 CUP	5	1	1	1
	1.5 CUPS	8	2	1	1
	2 CUPS	10	2	1	1
ONIONS, CHOPPED	1/2 CUP	34	8	1	7
	1 CUP	67	16	2	14
	1.5 CUPS	100	24	3	21
	2 CUPS	134	32	4	28
RADISHES	1/2 CUP	10	2	1	1
	1 CUP	19	4	2	2
	1.5 CUPS	29	6	3	3
	2 CUPS	38	8	4	4

Quick Glance MACRO BREAKDOWN

Veggies

	SERVING SIZE	CALORIES	GRAMS TOTAL CARBS	GRAMS FIBER	NET CARBS
SPINACH	1/2 CUP	4	6	0	0
	1 CUP	7	1	1	0
	1.5 CUPS	11	7	1	1
	2 CUPS	14	2	1	1
TOMATO	1/2 CUP	16	4	1	2
	1 CUP	32	7	2	5
	1.5 CUPS	48	11	3	7
	2 CUPS	64	14	4	10
TOMATOES, CHERRY	1/2 CUP	14	3	1	2
	1 CUP	27	6	2	4
	1.5 CUPS	41	9	3	6
	2 CUPS	54	12	4	8

OFF PROTOCOL Veggies

	SERVING SIZE	CALORIES	TOTAL CARBS	GRAMS FIBER	NET CARBS
BELL PEPPER	1/2 CUP	23	5	3	3
	1 CUP	46	9	3	6
	1.5 CUPS	69	14	5	9
	2 CUPS	92	18	6	12
BROCCOLI	1/2 CUP	16	3	1	2
	1 CUP	31	6	2	4
	1.5 CUPS	47	9	4	5
	2 CUPS	93	18	7	11
CROOKNECK SQUASH	1/2 CUP	13	3	1	1
	1 CUP	25	5	3	3
	1.5 CUPS	38	8	4	4
	2 CUPS	75	16	8	8

Quick Glance MACRO BREAKDOWN

OFF PROTOCOL Veggies	SERVING SIZE	CALORIES	TOTAL CARBS	GRAMS FIBER	NET CARBS
MUSHROOMS, SLICES	1/2 CUP	8	1	0	1
	1 CUP	15	2	1	2
	1.5 CUPS	23	3	1	3
	2 CUPS	45	7	2	4
ZUCCHINI, CHOPPED	1/2 CUP	10	2	1	1
	1 CUP	20	4	1	3
	1.5 CUPS	30	6	2	4
	2 CUPS	60	12	4	8
OTHER					
OTHER					
OTHER					
OTHER					

Your Humble **INDEX**

Thanks to Victoria of Oregon...an hCGer in my audience who noticed a glaring problem - my book did not originally have an index. Duh!! Thanks for your feedback and tips on creating it!

LINKS/BOOKS/OTHER COOL INTERNET STUFF:

HCGCHICA'S SOCIAL MEDIA:

Facebook, Instagram: hcgchica
Pinterest, Twitter: hcgchica (surprise!)
Email: hcgchica@hcgchica.com

SANITY SAVERS ON THE HCG DIET:

- hcgchica.com/hcgsanity
- hcgchica.com/cookbooks
- hcgchica.com/hcgbooks

- hCG Diet Gourmet Cookbooks - *Tammy Skye*
- Weight Loss Apocalypse - Emotional Eating Rehab Through the hCG Protocol - *Robin Woodall*

HORMONE STUFF:

Links

- hcgchica.com/hormonelinks
- hcgchica.com/findadoc
- Stopthethyroidmadness.com
- Jeffreydachmd.com

Books
(find the links to these books at hcgchica.com/hormonelinks)
- Stop the Thyroid Madness - *Janie A. Bowthorpe*

- Iodine - Why You Need It, Why You Can't Live Without It - *David Brownstein, M.D.*
- Hypothyroidism - Type 2 - *Mark Starr, M.D.*
- Recovering with T3 - My Journey from Hypothyroidism to Good Health Using the T3 Thyroid Hormone - *Paul Robinson*
- Safe Uses of Cortisol - *William Jeffries*
- Bioidentical Hormones 101 - *Jeffrey Dach, M.D.*

OTHER LINKS IN BOOK:

- hcgchica.com/p2workbook - *workbook tutorial*
- hcgchica.com/mystory - *my personal before and after hCG weight loss story*
- hcgchica.com/loading - *phase 1 info*
- hcgchica.com/dosage - *details on hCG Dosage*
- hcgchica.com/sleep - *troubleshooting sleep*
- hcgchica.com/timing - *timing of rounds*
- hcgchica.com/noodles - *miracle noodles*
- hcgchica.com/p3 - *phase 3*
- p3tolife.com - *program for Phase 3*
- hcgchica.com/p4 - *phase 4*

Made in the USA
San Bernardino, CA
04 September 2017